I0449372

Sensual Synergy

The Intersection of
Health and Desire

By
Emma Blake

Copyright 2024 Lars Meiertoberens. All rights reserved.

No part of this book may be reproduced in any form or by any electronic or mechanical means including information storage and retrieval systems, without permission in writing from the author. The only exception is by a reviewer, who may quote short excerpts in a review.

Although the author and publisher have made every effort to ensure that the information in this book was correct at press time, the author and publisher do not assume and hereby disclaim any liability to any party for any loss, damage, or disruption caused by errors or omissions, whether such errors or omissions result from negligence, accident, or any other cause.

This publication is designed to provide accurate and authoritative information with regard to the subject matter covered. It is sold with the understanding that the publisher is not engaged in rendering professional services. If legal advice or other expert assistance is required, the services of a competent professional should be sought.

The fact that an organization or website is referred to in this work as a citation and/or a potential source of further information does not mean that the author or the publisher endorses the information the organization or website may provide or recommendations it may make.

Please remember that Internet websites listed in this work may have changed or disappeared between when this work was written and when it is read.

Sensual Synergy

The Intersection of
Health and Desire

Table of Contents

Introduction 1

Chapter 1: Understanding Sexual Health 5
    The Basics of Sexual Health.. 5
    How Sexual Health Influences Well-being.......................... 8

Chapter 2: Historical Perspectives on Sexual Desire 11
    Ancient Views on Desire and Health................................. 11
    Modern Perspectives and Shifts 14

Chapter 3: The Science Behind Sexual Energy 18
    What is Sexual Energy? 18
    The Physiology of Sexual Arousal...................................... 20

Chapter 4: Emotional Wellness and Sexuality 23
    Emotional Intimacy and Desire... 23
    Managing Emotional Blocks to Sexual Health 26

Chapter 5: Mental Health and Sexual Expression 29
    Exploring Psychological Barriers 29
    The Role of Mindfulness in Sexual Health 32

Chapter 6: Social Influences on Sexual Well-being 36
    Cultural Norms and Their Impact 36
    Navigating Relationships and Expectations 39

Chapter 7: Nutrition and Sexual Vitality........................... 42
    Foods that Fuel Desire 42
    The Connection Between Diet and Libido 45

Chapter 8: Physical Fitness and Sexual Health 49
    Exercise for Enhancing Sexual Well-being 49
    Yoga and Its Benefits for Desire 52

Chapter 9: Harnessing Erotic Energy for Health 56
    Techniques for Cultivating Sexual Energy 56
    The Healing Power of Eroticism 59

Chapter 10: Communication and Desire 62
    Effective Communication Skills for Intimacy 62
    Understanding and Sharing Desires 65

Chapter 11: Hormones and Sexual Function 68
    The Role of Hormones in Desire 68
    Balancing Hormones Naturally 71

Chapter 12: Exploring Sexual Identity 75
    The Spectrum of Sexual Identities 75
    Embracing One's Sexual Self 79

Chapter 13: Ageing and Sexuality 83
    Maintaining Desire Across the Lifespan 83
    Overcoming Age-related Challenges 86

Chapter 14: Overcoming Sexual Dysfunction 90
    Common Sexual Disorders and Their Solutions 90
    Mental Approaches to Healing Dysfunction 93

Chapter 15: Spiritual Aspects of Sexuality 97
    The Connection between Sexuality and Spirituality 97
    Practices for Spiritual Sexual Intimacy 100

Chapter 16: Creating a Pleasure- positive Mindset 104
    Shifting Perspectives on Pleasure 104
    Cultivating a Positive Sexual Outlook 107

Chapter 17: The Role of Sleep in Sexual Health 111
    Sleep's Impact on Desire and Performance 111

Improving Sleep for Better Sexual Health 114

Chapter 18: Managing Stress for Better Sex................................. 118
The Effects of Stress on Desire 118
Techniques for Stress Reduction 121

Chapter 19: Innovative Therapies for Sexual Wellness 125
Exploring Alternative Therapies 125
The Future of Sexual Care.. 128

Chapter 20: Embracing Change and Growth............................... 132
Adapting to Life Stages.. 132
Personal Growth through Sexual Exploration 135

Chapter 21: Establishing Boundaries in Sexual Relationships.......... 138
Recognising and Setting Boundaries.. 138
Respect and Consent in Sexual Interactions 142

Chapter 22: The Intersection of Technology and Sexuality 145
The Impact of Digital Platforms on Desire 145
Balancing Technology Use with Intimacy................................ 149

Chapter 23: Enhancing Desire Through Creativity 152
The Power of Creative Expression 152
Strategies for Keeping Desire Alive 156

Chapter 24: Building a Supportive Sexual Community 159
Finding Allies in Sexual Exploration 159
The Benefits of Community and Shared Experience................ 163

Chapter 25: Achieving Sexual Synergy....................................... 166
Integrating Sexual Health into Daily Life................................ 166
Creating a Harmonious Balance Between Health and Desire 169

Conclusion 172

Appendix A: Appendix.. 175

Introduction

In a world that often compartmentalises aspects of health and well-being, the pivotal role of sexual health tends to be overlooked or shrouded in taboo. Yet, our sexual selves are intricately woven into the fabric of our overall well-being, influencing not just our physical health but also our emotional, psychological, and social lives. Within these pages, we aim to illuminate this profound connection and provide insights into how embracing one's sexual health can lead to a more balanced and fulfilling life.

At first glance, sexual health might appear to be a distinct domain, separate from other facets of life. However, it's an essential part of who we are, an undercurrent that shapes our identity and impacts our health in multifaceted ways. Whether you're embarking on a journey of personal growth or seeking to enrich your relationships, understanding and integrating sexual health can unlock new levels of vitality and well-being.

Sexuality isn't just about the act itself; it encompasses a wide spectrum of desires, identities, energies, and expressions. It's about understanding your own needs, exploring the diverse range of human experiences, and finding meaningful connections with others. This book invites you to explore the richness of sexual health, encouraging you to see it not as an isolated experience but as a vibrant and integral part of being human.

The approach to sexual health presented here is inclusive and holistic. It acknowledges that our experiences and expressions of sexuality are influenced by a myriad of factors, including historical perspectives, cultural norms, emotional wellness, and even our diet and exercise regimens. By delving into these areas, you'll gain a greater understanding of how each aspect impacts the other and contributes to your overall health.

Our exploration begins with an understanding of the basics of sexual health and how it influences our well-being. From there, we'll journey through historical perspectives, considering how perceptions of desire have shifted from ancient times to the modern day. This historical lens helps unravel the complexities of our current understanding, providing insights into contemporary attitudes and beliefs.

We then dive into the science behind sexual energy and its physiological aspects. Sexual energy is often misunderstood or mystified, yet it's integral to our vitality. Recognising and harnessing this energy can lead to enhanced well-being and a deeper sense of connection with oneself and others.

Emotional wellness plays a pivotal role in how we experience and express our sexuality. Emotional intimacy, the building of deep, trusted bonds, is fundamental in fostering healthy sexual relationships. But navigating emotional blocks can be challenging, and understanding these barriers is key to unlocking greater sexual health.

Similarly, mental health is deeply interconnected with sexual expression. Psychological barriers can inhibit desire and sexual confidence. Yet, through practices such as mindfulness, individuals can cultivate a more profound awareness of both their minds and bodies, leading to a more fulfilling sexual life.

Social influences, including cultural and societal norms, shape our views and experiences of sexuality. Navigating these influences requires a delicate balance between respecting cultural contexts and expressing individual desires. By fostering open and honest communication, individuals can better navigate these complexities, creating relationships built on mutual understanding and respect.

Physical aspects such as nutrition and fitness can't be ignored when discussing sexual vitality. There is a noted synergy between what we consume, how we move, and our sexual energies. By being mindful of dietary choices and incorporating physical activities such as exercise and yoga, one can enhance libido and overall sexual well-being.

As we look further into holistic practices, you'll discover how erotic energy can be harnessed for healing and personal development. Techniques for cultivating this energy encourage reconnection with your body and its innate wisdom, allowing for transformative experiences.

One cannot overlook the importance of communication in intimate relationships. Understanding and articulating desires, practicing consent, and establishing boundaries are crucial components of healthy sexual interactions. This section will equip you with the skills to foster more profound connections with your partner(s), enhancing mutual satisfaction and intimacy.

Hormonal influences also play a significant role in desire. Fluctuations in hormones can greatly affect sexual function, yet through natural methods, one can work towards a balanced hormonal state, improving both health and sexual vitality.

In our ever-evolving understanding of identity, it's essential to explore the spectrum of sexual identities. Embracing one's sexual identity is a journey of self-discovery that enriches our understanding and acceptance of others' journeys. This acceptance fuels a truer, more authentic expression of self, enriching both personal and collective experiences.

As we navigate life's stages, sexual needs and desires inevitably evolve. Ageing doesn't mean the decline of sexual vitality; rather, it presents opportunities to redefine and adapt one's sexual expression. By embracing these changes, individuals can maintain a vibrant sexual life throughout their years.

This book also addresses common sexual dysfunctions and presents both mental and practical approaches to overcoming them. Thoughtful strategies empower individuals to seek solutions that align with their unique needs, fostering resilience and recovery.

Tapping into the spiritual aspects of sexuality offers profound insights. This exploration encourages an understanding of sexuality as a spiritual practice, helping deepen connections and enhance pleasure within sacred partnerships.

Shifting perspectives on pleasure, adopting a pleasure-positive mindset, and understanding the role of sleep and stress further contribute to one's sexual health. Innovative therapies present new horizons in sexual wellness, offering alternatives that are both exciting and empowering.

Ultimately, this journey is about embracing change, growth, and the continuous evolution of one's sexual self. The integration of sexual health into daily life promises more than just improved relationships; it leads to holistic growth and profound personal satisfaction.

By building a supportive community, whether through shared experiences or finding like-minded allies, individuals can find comfort and encouragement in their explorations. The power of creative expression further fuels desire, keeping relationships alive and thriving.

As you delve deeper into the book, consider every chapter as a stepping stone towards achieving sexual synergy. Through personal reflection and the practical tools shared, you will be equipped to create a harmonious balance between health and desire.

Chapter 1:
Understanding Sexual Health

Sexual health, often intertwined with both joy and complexity, is a crucial aspect of our overall well-being that demands more attention and understanding. By delving into the fundamentals, we uncover how it goes beyond mere physical acts, encompassing emotional, mental, and social dimensions that coalesce to form an integral part of who we are. The interplay between our sexual health and well-being forms a synergy that reverberates through our lives, potentially enhancing relationships and enriching personal growth. In this journey, recognising the significance of sexual health opens pathways to not only experiencing greater fulfilment but also empowering ourselves to take control of our own narratives. It's about embracing a balanced approach where knowledge and awareness lead to enriched life experiences, unlocking a fullness that spills over into every aspect of our existence.

The Basics of Sexual Health

Understanding the fundamentals of sexual health is central to embracing a fulfilling and balanced life. At its core, sexual health isn't just about the absence of disease or dysfunction; it's about recognising and celebrating a vital aspect of human experience that contributes significantly to our overall well-being. It's an avenue through which intimacy, pleasure, and identity can be explored, contributing to personal empowerment and life satisfaction.

Sexual health encompasses a range of physical, emotional, and social factors. It's about knowing who you are, understanding your desires, and confidently communicating them. This process involves accepting your body and its functions, fostering healthy relationships, and making informed decisions about sexual behaviours. By doing so, individuals not only enhance their own lives but also contribute to a more inclusive and understanding society.

One can't underestimate the importance of education in sexual health. It goes beyond the basic lessons of biology to address broader themes, including consent, respect, and emotional connection. Comprehensive sexual education empowers individuals to make choices that align with their values and desires. Informative resources encourage open discussions and dispel myths, cultivating a positive and realistic approach to sexual health.

Another pillar of sexual health is personal empowerment. Feeling empowered involves taking ownership of one's sexual health, understanding risks, and navigating relationships safely and respectfully. It's about advocating for oneself, setting boundaries, and understanding consent deeply. When individuals feel empowered in their sexual health, they are more likely to engage in healthy behaviors and enjoy fulfilling intimate relationships.

It's equally crucial to address the emotional and psychological facets of sexual health. Sexuality is intimately connected with emotions which can add depth to relationships. By recognising emotional needs and articulating them, individuals can deepen connections, build trust, and foster mutual satisfaction. Emotional intelligence plays a significant role in sexual health, facilitating understanding and cooperation between partners.

Social influences also play an integral role. They shape perceptions, inform behaviours, and form societal norms. Understanding the pressures and expectations from society helps individuals navigate their sexual identity and behaviours with greater clarity and confidence. By acknowledging social influences, one can challenge stereotypes and advocate for a healthier dialogue around sexuality.

Physical health is undeniably interconnected with sexual well-being. Regular exercise, a balanced diet, and sufficient rest enhance not just physical vitality, but also libido and sexual performance. It's essential to view physical health and sexual health as two sides of the same coin — each affecting the other in profound ways that enhance one's quality of life.

An important aspect, often overlooked, is the role of mental health in sexual well-being. Stress, anxiety, and depression can diminish libido and hinder sexual function. Promoting mental health and employing techniques like mindfulness can improve not only general well-being but also create a healthy environment for sexual exploration and intimacy.

Communication remains a keystone of healthy sexual relationships. Expressing desires, boundaries, and expectations openly with a partner fosters an environment of trust and mutual respect. It's through communication that misunderstandings can be resolved and deeper connections formed, paving the way for more meaningful interactions.

Finally, cultivating a positive and open mindset towards sexuality is essential. By challenging negative beliefs and embracing a healthier perspective, individuals open themselves up to richer experiences. Emphasising pleasure, understanding, and growth over mere functionality leads to a more integrated and fulfilling experience of one's sexual self.

In summary, the basics of sexual health provide a crucial foundation for leading a balanced and fulfilling life. They intertwine with every aspect of our being, influencing how we connect with ourselves and others. By understanding and valuing the multifaceted nature of sexual health, individuals can build a harmonious life enriched by deeper intimacy, greater personal insight, and enhanced well-being.

How Sexual Health Influences Well-being

Sexual health plays a pivotal role in shaping our overall well-being, influencing both our physical vitality and emotional resilience. It acts as a compass guiding us toward a more fulfilling life, where joy and satisfaction aren't mere afterthoughts but rather essential components of our everyday existence. Understanding how sexual health interweaves with various aspects of well-being can transform our approach to both ourselves and our relationships.

Firstly, let's consider the physical implications. Sexual health impacts numerous bodily systems—from cardiovascular health to hormonal balance. Engaging in sexual activity can stimulate the release of hormones such as oxytocin and endorphins, which promote feelings of happiness and contentment. Improved circulation and cardiovascular health are often associated with a regular and healthy sexual life, linking sexual satisfaction directly to overall physical fitness.

Moreover, sexual health isn't just about the act itself but encompasses a broader range of intimate activities and connections. Whether it's touch, intimacy, or simply being comfortable in one's own skin, these components foster a sense of physical well-being. When practiced in a healthy, consensual manner, sexual activities can enhance our psychological health too. They help in reducing stress, combating anxiety, and even promoting better sleep—elements crucial for maintaining mental and physical balance.

On an emotional level, sexual health can significantly influence our sense of self and connectedness with others. A healthy sexual identity and expression can bolster self-esteem and confidence. For many, the ability to explore and understand their sexual desires and boundaries can lead to deeper self-awareness and personal growth. Stronger emotional connections often develop alongside sexual intimacy, building trust and an emotional bond between partners that is vital for long-term relationship satisfaction.

In relationships, sexual health acts as a pillar, supporting open communication and mutual respect. When partners can openly discuss their desires, boundaries, and even fears, it creates an environment of trust and honesty. This openness leads to stronger, more resilient partnerships. The mutual exploration of sexual health can even reignite passion and connection in relationships that may feel stagnant or strained.

However, challenges in sexual health can also highlight areas needing attention and growth. Sexual dysfunction or a disconnect between partners can serve as crucial indicators of underlying issues, whether they be emotional, psychological, or physical. Addressing these challenges head-on can be an empowering process, leading to significant personal and relational development.

Sexual health also interacts intriguingly with our mental well-being. Practices that foster mindfulness and presence—often essential components of satisfying sexual experiences—can anchor us in the present, reducing the noise of anxiety and past regrets. The focus required during sexual experiences encourages a mindfulness that can ripple out into other areas of life, teaching us how to be more present and engaged in everyday moments.

In the tapestry of our well-being, sexual health is a thread that ties together various facets of human experience. It reminds us that pleasure is not just a transient experience but a meaningful part of a complete life. When embraced fully and healthily, sexual health encourages a life filled with vitality and resilience, underscoring the notion that our happiness is closely linked to how we express and engage with our sexual selves.

While sexual health undoubtedly contributes to individual well-being, it also plays a role in creating healthier communities. A society that encourages open dialogue about sexual health and respects individual sexual rights tends to be more empathetic and equitable. When communities support diverse expressions of sexuality and respect consensual relationships, they become safer and more nurturing environments for individuals to explore and express their sexual selves freely.

The influence of sexual health on well-being is multifaceted, touching upon our physical, emotional, and social spheres. Understanding and embracing this connection fosters a holistic sense of health and satisfaction that permeates all aspects of life, reminding us that sexual well-being is not an isolated component but a vital piece of the well-being puzzle. Engaging with our sexual health can empower us to live fuller, more integrated lives where balance and happiness are within reach.

Chapter 2:
Historical Perspectives
on Sexual Desire

Throughout history, human societies have been profoundly shaped by their perceptions of sexual desire. From the ancient civilisations that intertwined eroticism with health and spirituality to modern shifts that recognise a diverse landscape of desires, the tapestry of human experience reveals a constant evolution. In early cultures, sexuality was often revered as a divine force, vital to both individual well-being and communal prosperity. These ancient views laid a foundation, though over time, cultural attitudes towards desire have frequently oscillated between liberation and repression. As we progressed into more contemporary eras, sexual desire was not only medicalised but also subjected to societal norms, reflecting the changing dynamics of power, morality, and personal freedom. Understanding these historical contexts enriches our present-day exploration, offering insightful reflections on how attitudes towards sexual desire can illuminate pathways to a balanced and fulfilling life. This journey through time underscores the undeniable link between embracing our desires and achieving overall well-being, empowering us to acknowledge and integrate this vital aspect of who we are.

Ancient Views on Desire and Health

In the tapestry of human history, sexuality and desire have been both revered and questioned, perceived as cornerstones of vitality, health, and harmony. Ancient civilisations possessed profound insights into the relationship between sexual desire and overall health, often intertwining these notions with their broader philosophical and spiritual frameworks. The past reveals a fascinating mosaic of beliefs that can inspire contemporary understandings of sexuality, health, and well-being.

In Ancient Greece, the concept of desire was integral to discussions about health and the human condition. Greek physicians and philosophers like Hippocrates and Plato considered sexual activity essential to maintaining balance within the body. Hippocrates, often dubbed the "Father of Medicine," believed that sexual activity contributed to the regulation of bodily humours, which were thought to influence emotions and physical health. A balanced sexual life was seen as part of a responsible approach to personal health, serving as a control mechanism for excessive desires that could otherwise lead to imbalance and illness.

Meanwhile, Plato's philosophies introduced a more nuanced understanding of desire. By distinguishing between physical desire and a higher form of love or "Eros," he highlighted the multifaceted nature of desire, arguing for its importance in achieving personal and spiritual growth. Herein lies an early recognition of how sexual desire intertwined with emotional and spiritual health, a concept still mirrored in today's holistic health perspectives.

In the Indian subcontinent, sexual desire and health were extensively explored and documented in ancient texts such as the *Kama Sutra* and the *Ayurvedic* treatises. The *Kama Sutra*, much more than an ancient manual on sexual positions, offered a comprehensive guide on living a balanced life, underscoring the significance of desire in achieving harmony in human relationships. It advocated for sexual health as part of one's overall well-being, promoting practices that enhanced vitality and contentment.

Ayurveda, the ancient Indian system of medicine, provided a sophisticated understanding of how sexual health affects physical and mental states. According to Ayurvedic principles, sexual energy is a powerful life force, known as "Shakti," which, when harnessed correctly, could invigorate and sustain the body. Ayurveda emphasises the impact of lifestyle, diet, and sexual practices on maintaining "Ojas," the vital life energy responsible for health and longevity, recognising the crucial role of balanced sexual expression in achieving holistic health.

In ancient China, sexuality was embedded within the broader philosophical context of Taoism, which presented a unique view of health and longevity. Taoists considered sexual energy or "jing" to be a vital essence that should be cultivated and preserved. Maintaining a harmonious balance between yin and yang energies, often mirrored through sexual practices, was seen as essential to sustaining life and enhancing spiritual development. Practices like "dual cultivation," integrating sexual energy for spiritual growth, signified a deep interconnection between desire and both physical and metaphysical health.

Sexuality in ancient Egypt carried spiritual significance as well. The ancient Egyptians perceived sexual desire as crucial not merely for procreation but as a divine force that could both heal and enhance life's pleasures. Their mythology frequently illustrated sexual themes, showcasing how desire and health were honoured as sacred bonds between humans and gods. The reverence for fertility and sexual rituals demonstrated an acknowledgment of desire as a foundational force for creation and rejuvenation.

Furthermore, the connection between desire and health is evident in ancient Mesopotamia, where sexual and fertility deities played pivotal roles in the health and prosperity of communities. Temples dedicated to goddesses like Inanna or Ishtar were centres not only for worship but also for healing, suggesting an intrinsic link between spiritual devotion, sexual health, and societal well-being.

As we delve deeper into these historical perspectives, it becomes apparent that sexuality wasn't merely a biological or hedonistic pursuit in ancient times. Instead, it was enveloped in cultural, moral, and spiritual dimensions. Many ancient societies seemed to understand that a balanced sexual life was integral to achieving not just personal happiness but also contributing to the welfare and continuity of the community.

The perspectives on desire and health from ancient civilisations offer poignant lessons for today's discourse on sexual well-being. They remind us that embracing our sexuality can be a profound pathway toward achieving a balanced, fulfilling life. By looking back at these ancient teachings, we can glean insights into how the integration of desire and health within a broader spiritual and philosophical context can enrich our understanding of human wellness and happiness.

Thus, while the cosmologies of these civilisations may differ, a common thread emerges: desire was not an enemy of health, but an ally. Whether through religious rituals, medicinal practices, or philosophical musings, it is recognised as a vital part of human existence, just as breathing is. Revisiting these ancient ideas can provide a rich source of wisdom as we seek to embrace and integrate sexual health into our modern lives.

Modern Perspectives and Shifts

The landscape of sexual desire has witnessed significant shifts over the decades. Once confined to the shadows of taboo and discretion, sexual desire now sits at the intersection of cultural dialogue and personal empowerment. Modern perspectives on sexual desire reflect a complex tapestry woven from scientific advancements, changing societal norms, and a growing emphasis on personal wellness.

In recent years, the conversation around sexual desire has expanded beyond heteronormative frameworks, embracing a more inclusive understanding of sexuality that acknowledges diverse orientations and expressions. This inclusivity is not just about recognising differences but celebrating them. The expansion incorporates a multitude of identities, from LGBTQ+ communities actively shaping the discourse to the increasing visibility of non-binary and fluid identities, each calling for the acknowledgment of their unique experiences and needs.

One cannot overlook the role of technology in reshaping how individuals perceive and experience sexual desire. Dating apps and online platforms have transformed courtship rituals, often accelerating the pace at which intimacy develops. While this digital transformation has created opportunities for connection and exploration, it also presents challenges, such as navigating authenticity and fostering genuine connections in digital environments. These platforms have democratised access to potential partners, while simultaneously raising questions about privacy and consent in a digital age.

Moreover, scientific research has brought unprecedented insights into the biological and psychological mechanisms of sexual desire, offering evidence-based pathways for enhancing individual and relational well-being. Contemporary studies delve into the complexities of libido, exploring not just hormonal influences but also the impacts of mental health, stress, and lifestyle choices. Understanding these dynamics allows individuals to take a more active role in managing their sexual health, recognising that physical and emotional wellness significantly influence desire.

A striking modern shift is the decoupling of sexual desire from traditional narratives of reproduction. The focus is increasingly on sexual pleasure and its crucial role in emotional and physical health. Sex-positive movements advocate for a mindset that views sexual expression as a fundamental human experience, essential for individual fulfilment. This paradigm shift encourages the cultivation of pleasure as an integral aspect of a healthy lifestyle, challenging historical views that often relegated sex solely to the realm of procreation.

Equally important is the conversation about consent and autonomy, reshaped by modern social movements. The #MeToo era has placed a spotlight on issues of power dynamics and mutual respect in sexual encounters. These discussions have brought about necessary and overdue changes in legal and cultural arenas, prompting critical introspection and reform. Consent is now recognised as an ongoing, enthusiastic process, reinforcing the need for communication and negotiation between partners.

The integration of mindfulness into sexual wellness practices represents another noteworthy shift. Mindfulness encourages a present-focused approach, facilitating deeper connections with one's body and emotions. By fostering a non-judgmental awareness, mindfulness practices help individuals overcome anxieties, enhance pleasure, and nurture intimacy. This holistic perspective aligns sexual desire with overall well-being, promoting a balanced and thoughtful approach to sexual health.

In tandem with these innovations, societal perspectives on gender roles continue to evolve. Traditional gender norms are increasingly challenged, allowing individuals greater freedom to express themselves authentically without the constraints of outdated stereotypes. This fluidity extends to sexual expression, inviting exploration and sincerity in a society that increasingly values personal truth over prescriptive norms.

The modern era also witnesses a surge in sexual education reform, aimed at providing comprehensive and inclusive information to individuals of all ages. Unlike past, limited models of sexual education, today's curricula increasingly address topics such as consent, diverse sexualities, and emotional health, equipping individuals with the knowledge to make informed choices about their sexual lives. Education empowers individuals, breaking cycles of ignorance and stigma, thereby fostering healthy relationships grounded in understanding and respect.

Furthermore, personal empowerment and individual agency remain at the heart of modern shifts in sexual desire. Individuals are encouraged to define their desires and boundaries, asserting their needs within relationships. This empowerment is a departure from historical tendencies of silence and submission, advocating instead for assertive and confident participation in one's sexual narrative.

While these modern perspectives and shifts provide opportunities for growth and fulfilment, they also challenge individuals to critically engage with their beliefs and behaviours surrounding sexual desire. As people increasingly embrace a holistic view of sexual health, they are encouraged to reflect on the multifaceted influences on their desire and to seek harmony between their emotional, physical, and relational selves.

This contemporary understanding inspires a more nuanced dialogue that respects tradition while embracing evolution, merging ancient wisdom with modern science. Ultimately, these shifts not only redefine what it means to experience and express sexual desire but also pave the way for deeper connections and more fulfilling relationships, enhancing the quality of life for individuals and communities alike.

Chapter 3:
The Science Behind Sexual Energy

Sexual energy—it's more than just the spark that fuels romantic passion. It's a vibrant force deeply embedded in our physiology, playing a crucial role in the dynamic between our bodies and minds. At its core, sexual energy is about the interconnectedness of our sexes with our overall vitality, linking physical health with emotional and mental wellness. Underlying this powerful connection is a dance of hormones, neurotransmitters, and physical responses that illuminate the pathways to pleasure and intimacy. By understanding this energy's scientific foundation, we can unlock its potential, allowing us to harness it not merely for procreation or fleeting enjoyment but as a fundamental pillar of our well-being. Embracing the science behind sexual energy offers us the tools to enrich our lives, foster deeper connections, and tap into a source of profound personal empowerment, driving us toward a more fulfilled existence.

What is Sexual Energy?

Sexual energy, often referred to as life force energy in various philosophical and spiritual traditions, is a vital force that not only drives sexual desire but also influences our overall health and well-being. Imagine it as a current, flowing through the human body and mind, fuelling creativity, joy, and a sense of fulfilment. This energy isn't just about physical attraction or the act of sex – it encompasses emotional, mental, and spiritual realms, linking deeply to who we are and how we connect with others.

At the physiological level, sexual energy is closely tied to hormones and the nervous system. When aroused, our bodies undergo a cascade of hormonal changes that not only prepare us for sexual activity but also enhance mood and bolster immune function. This physiological response demonstrates a natural interplay between pleasure and health, highlighting how sexual energy can have far-reaching effects beyond the bedroom.

While the physiological aspects are significant, it's crucial to look beyond the physical. Sexual energy embodies an emotional and psychological component that's intimately connected to our sense of self. This energy can invigorate personal exploration, helping us to understand our desires and how they fit into the wider tapestry of our lives. By acknowledging and cultivating this energy, we can potentially unlock a heightened state of joy and personal growth.

The concept of sexual energy isn't confined to modern science; it appears throughout history across diverse cultures. Many ancient traditions view it as a sacred energy, one that merits respect and understanding. For instance, in tantric teachings, sexual energy is seen as a powerful force for spiritual awakening, capable of transcending the physical and connecting individuals with the divine. Such perspectives offer insight into the depth and breadth of influence that sexual energy can wield.

Psychologically, harnessing sexual energy can contribute significantly to our mental health. In a world fraught with stress and anxiety, tapping into the vitality of sexual energy can offer a sanctuary of peace and strength. It encourages a profound connection with oneself, fostering resilience and self-assurance. These positive mental states can, in turn, improve interpersonal relationships and enhance life satisfaction.

Moreover, sexual energy can be a catalyst for creativity. Many artists, writers, and innovators have spoken of the inspiration derived from this wellspring of energy, suggesting that tapping into one's sexual energy can lead to bursts of creativity and new ideas. This makes sense when considering the interconnectedness of the brain's pleasure and reward systems, which light up during both sexual arousal and creative activities.

Understanding sexual energy also means acknowledging its role in personal relationships. The energy ignites and sustains intimacy, enabling partners to connect on multiple levels. In healthy relationships, sexual energy is often the glue that binds people together, nurturing connections that are both deep and fulfilling. It's through the exchange of this energy that partnerships can grow richer and more meaningful.

On the flip side, when sexual energy is stifled or misdirected, it can lead to frustration, dissatisfaction, or even health issues. Recognising how this energy manifests in our lives is crucial for maintaining harmony. Just as any other form of energy, sexual energy requires balance and flow, benefiting not just sexual health but overall well-being.

In conclusion, sexual energy is a multifaceted phenomenon encompassing physical, emotional, mental, and spiritual aspects of the human experience. It is a dynamic force, capable of driving creative expression and transforming our physical and emotional landscapes. By understanding and nurturing this energy, individuals can enhance their health, deepen intimacy, and find greater joy in life.

The Physiology of Sexual Arousal

The intricate dance of sexual arousal begins in the mind and flows through the body, intertwining complex networks of neurological, physiological, and emotional responses. Understanding the physiology of sexual arousal provides us with valuable insights into our own bodies and the interconnectedness of our mind and health. This section will delve into the fundamental components that trigger the arousal process, revealing the natural wonders of our sexual physiology.

Sexual arousal starts with desire, often initiated by stimuli that vary widely from person to person. These stimuli can be visual, auditory, or even imaginative. Our senses play a crucial role in sending signals to the brain. The brain acts as the command centre, interpreting these signals and setting off a cascade of reactions. The hypothalamus, a key player in this process, interacts with various neurotransmitters like dopamine, which are pivotal in the pleasure and reward systems. These brain chemicals surge, creating the anticipated pleasurable sensations and increasing feelings of arousal.

As the brain processes these signals, the body responds in kind. One can't overlook the role of the autonomic nervous system, which steers the physiological changes through its two branches: the sympathetic and parasympathetic systems. Initially, the parasympathetic nervous system triggers an increase in blood flow to the genital area, leading to the physical signs of arousal. For individuals with vulvas, this means the engorgement and lubrication of the vaginal area. For those with penises, the result is an erection.

These physiological changes involve the dilation of blood vessels and a complex interplay of hormones and enzymes. Nitric oxide is released, relaxing the vascular smooth muscles and enhancing blood flow, which, in turn, maintains genital arousal. However, the process is not only confined to the genital area. The entire body becomes attuned to the arousal state, with increased heart rate, heightened senses, and mild sweating—all painting a picture of the body's total readiness.

Moreover, sexual arousal is accompanied by changes in other bodily systems as well. Endocrine responses include the secretion of hormones like oestrogen and testosterone, which further fuel sexual drive. Meanwhile, the respiratory rate increases, preparing the body for the physical exertion that may follow during sexual activity. It's a comprehensive system of responses that illustrates how arousal transpires, from the brain's initial signal to the body's full physical engagement.

It's essential to recognise that each individual's experience of arousal is unique. Hormonal variations, psychological state, health, and even past experiences can influence how one's body reacts. Factors such as stress, anxiety, or fatigue can inhibit these natural processes, showcasing the delicate balance required for sexual arousal to occur harmoniously. Understanding these nuances can inspire individuals to cultivate a heartfelt awareness and appreciation for their singular arousal journey.

Furthermore, the complexities of arousal demonstrate its significance not only in sexual health but also in emotional and relational well-being. Arousal is interwoven with emotional experience, and emotional intimacy can enhance or diminish the physiological responses. Recognising the link between emotional states and physical arousal emphasises the importance of addressing both body and mind in discussions of sexual health.

Finally, cultivating an understanding of the physiology behind arousal is an empowering tool—one that aids individuals in taking charge of their sexual health. With this knowledge, one can better navigate arousal in its many forms, whether during solo exploration or shared experiences, fostering greater intimacy and satisfaction in life. Embracing this aspect of our health leads to a deeper connection with oneself and with others, steering us towards a more holistic, balanced life.

Chapter 4:
Emotional Wellness and Sexuality

Emotional wellness and sexuality are deeply intertwined, forming a crucial foundation for a life that's both balanced and fulfilling. When emotional well-being is prioritized, it enhances one's ability to connect on intimate levels, fueling desire and intimacy in relationships. This connection goes beyond mere physical attraction, tapping into the profound sense of security and understanding that supports healthy sexual expression. Our capacity to be emotionally present can open doors to richer, more meaningful sexual experiences, shedding light on the importance of addressing emotional barriers that may hinder sexual health. By fostering emotional resilience and awareness, we allow our sexual selves to thrive, contributing to overall personal growth and harmony in our relationships. Embracing and nurturing this link empowers individuals to transform their intimate lives into dynamic expressions of their truest selves.

Emotional Intimacy and Desire

In the tapestry of human connection, emotional intimacy is the thread that binds individuals not just to each other, but to the deepest parts of themselves. It's the space where two people can be vulnerable and real, sharing their innermost thoughts and feelings without fear of judgment. This level of closeness acts as a powerful fuel for desire, weaving sexuality with emotion in a way that's both profound and transformative. But what exactly is the link between emotional intimacy and desire, and why does it hold such sway over our sexual well-being?

Let's start with emotional intimacy itself. It's more than just closeness; it's a feeling of connectedness that stems from shared experiences, mutual respect, and open communication. It's the art of being fully present, listening actively, and offering empathy. When emotional intimacy is cultivated, it opens the door to a deeper level of trust and understanding. This environment provides a safe haven where desires can flourish, and sexual energy can flow freely. In essence, emotional intimacy serves as both the groundwork and catalyst for sexual desire.

Desire, while often associated with physical attraction and arousal, is intrinsically linked to emotions. It thrives on the emotional connection between partners and is amplified when individuals feel seen, heard, and valued. When practitioners of intimacy engage both their hearts and minds, they create a blend of passion and compassion that can elevate physical encounters into something much more meaningful. Desire blooms best in an environment rich with emotional nuance and mutual appreciation.

Yet, establishing and maintaining emotional intimacy can be daunting. It demands vulnerability — a willingness to expose one's true self, complete with imperfections and fears. This honesty is where true intimacy begins, though it can feel unsettling at first. For many, the fear of vulnerability can be a barrier to achieving both emotional closeness and the heightened desire it engenders. The journey to dismantling these fears begins with self-awareness, accepting oneself fully, and recognising the reciprocal nature of intimacy.

In intimate partnerships, emotional intimacy is not a static achievement but a dynamic process. It requires continuous effort, attention, and nurturing. Regular communication and honest dialogue form the bedrock of this process. Expressing emotions openly, sharing dreams, and discussing fears are all integral parts. Couples who prioritize such exchanges often find their desires not only survive but thrive. This constant effort to remain emotionally connected ensures that the tie between intimacy and desire remains strong and unbroken.

It's crucial to consider that everyone experiences and expresses emotional intimacy differently. Factors such as cultural background, personal history, and previous relationship experiences shape how one approaches emotional closeness. Understanding these individual differences is essential in creating a harmonious connection. Learning to navigate these variances can foster a more personalised and satisfying relationship for both partners, leading to a flourishing of both emotional and sexual well-being.

The interplay of emotional intimacy and desire isn't isolated from other elements of life. Broader life responsibilities, stress, and external pressures can impact one's emotional landscape and subsequently, sexual desire. Balancing these elements requires mindfulness and intentional effort to prioritise the emotional aspects of the relationship. Recognising and managing these external pressures can help maintain a healthy and vibrant intimate connection.

For those searching to deepen their understanding of this intricate dance between emotion and desire, it might be helpful to engage with practices that promote self-reflection and emotional growth. Journaling, meditative practices, or even open dialogues with one's partner about each other's emotional needs can be enlightening. These practices encourage a more profound connection with oneself and, consequently, with one's partner, setting the stage for deeper emotional intimacy.

Ultimately, the sacred link between emotional intimacy and desire cannot be understated. It reminds us that sexuality is not merely a physical act but an expression of deeper emotional currents. When cultivated properly, these currents have the power to enrich relationships, enhance personal well-being, and create lives imbued with passion and affection. As we explore this powerful connection, we continually rediscover the potential for emotional intimacy to lead to greater fulfilment in our lives and relationship with sexuality.

Managing Emotional Blocks to Sexual Health

In the intricate tapestry of human health, sexual well-being holds a prominent thread that weaves through our emotional lives. Yet, the journey to harmonious sexual health is often impeded by emotional blocks that can stifle desire and intimacy. Understanding and overcoming these barriers is a crucial step towards a more fulfilling existence.

Emotional blocks to sexual health can manifest in countless ways, each unique to the individual experiencing them. They can root themselves in past traumas, negative self-perceptions, or unresolved emotional conflicts. These blocks, while challenging, are not insurmountable. By delving into their causes and addressing them with compassion and understanding, one can begin to dismantle the barriers that hinder sexual expression.

To begin exploring these emotional blocks, it is essential to acknowledge them without judgement. Self-awareness is the first, and often the most challenging, step. By recognising the specific emotions or past experiences that are creating obstacles, individuals can start charting a path to healthier sexual dynamics. Journaling, meditation, or speaking with a trusted confidant can often illuminate these hidden corners of the psyche.

Consider the role of self-talk; the internal dialogue that shapes much of how we perceive the world and ourselves within it. Negative self-talk, particularly about body image or sexual worthiness, can significantly impact sexual health. Challenging these destructive narratives with loving, affirming statements can begin to shift the internal landscape from one of criticism to acceptance and love.

However, it's not only past experiences or self-talk that can be culprits in creating emotional barriers. Societal pressures also play a significant role. Cultural norms can impose expectations and guilt, restricting sexual expression and exploration. Challenging these norms requires courage—choosing to craft one's own narrative around sexuality, uninfluenced by external dictates, can foster genuine sexual and emotional freedom.

The role of relationships in managing emotional blocks is profound. Trust and communication within intimate partnerships are pivotal in this process. Open dialogues about desires, fears, and boundaries create a safe space where emotional blocks can be explored and understood. Encouraging partners to support each other in their personal growth can transform relationships into a source of healing and strength rather than sources of pressure or insecurity.

Additionally, emotional blocks often thrive in isolation but diminish when brought into the light through shared experiences. Finding community, whether through support groups or workshops, can offer a sense of belonging and validation. Hearing others' stories can normalize personal struggles and provide new perspectives on handling emotional challenges related to sexual health.

Therapeutic approaches, such as cognitive behavioural therapy (CBT) or psychodynamic therapy, also offer structured ways to address and manage emotional blocks. They provide professional guidance and a framework for exploring emotions, helping to identify patterns of thought that hinder sexual well-being. Therapy offers a safe space for vulnerability, where individuals can process past traumas or current anxieties without fear of judgement.

As you navigate these emotional landscapes, it's vital to embrace a spirit of patience and kindness towards oneself. Growth, particularly personal growth revolving around deeply intimate aspects of life like sexuality, is rarely linear. It's a journey marked by small steps and occasional setbacks, but every move forward contributes to healing and liberation.

One practical strategy in managing emotional blocks is mindfulness. Practicing mindfulness during intimate moments, focusing on the present sensations rather than lingering on anxious thoughts, can help redirect energy towards pleasure and connection. Mindfulness not only enhances sexual experiences but also alleviates performance anxieties and negative self-perceptions, paving the way for more fulfilling and authentic interactions.

Transforming emotional blocks into stepping stones for better sexual health requires an intertwining of introspection, communication, and external support. By bravely confronting these barriers with openness and love, the path towards true sexual wellness comes into clear view. This journey of self-awareness and healing not only enriches sexual health but also holistically enhances emotional and mental well-being, encompassing the core of a balanced and joyous life.

Ultimately, the management of emotional blocks to sexual health is about embracing vulnerability and change. It is about reclaiming one's narrative and creating a personal definition of sexual health that aligns with one's deepest values and desires. Through understanding and addressing emotional blocks, individuals can transcend limitations, welcoming a more vibrant, integrated approach to their health and well-being.

Chapter 5:
Mental Health and
Sexual Expression

Mental health and sexual expression are deeply intertwined, shaping and influencing each other in a delicate dance. When we delve into the realm of sexual expression, we uncover a complex interplay of psychological factors that can either liberate or constrain our capacity to experience fulfilment. It's about recognising the psychological barriers—anxiety, depression or past traumas—that might hold us back from fully engaging in and enjoying our sexual selves. Through the lens of mindfulness and self-awareness, individuals can begin to break down these barriers, creating a space where mental health and sexuality coalesce harmoniously. Embracing this connection empowers us to assert agency over our sexual narrative, enhancing our well-being and fostering a more intimate connection with ourselves and others. This journey isn't just an exploration of desire but a transformative path to mental clarity and emotional resilience, encouraging a more nuanced and enriched experience of life's pleasures.

Exploring Psychological Barriers

Understanding the intricate relationship between mental health and sexual expression unveils a landscape teeming with psychological barriers. These barriers, often shaped by societal norms and personal experiences, can hinder one's ability to fully engage with their sexual identity, impacting overall well-being. Every individual's journey toward embracing their sexual self is unique, laden with its own set of challenges and breakthroughs.

One of the predominant psychological barriers is shame, a powerful emotion that can silently dictate our sexual expressions and experiences. Rooted in cultural, familial, or religious beliefs, shame can distort perceptions of what's acceptable or desirable, planting seeds of self-doubt. The struggle with such internalised shame can create a chasm between one's true desires and their expression, leading to a compromised sense of authenticity.

Moreover, fear, whether of judgement, rejection, or vulnerability, serves as a significant barrier to sexual expression. Fear instils a reluctance to explore or communicate one's desires, fostering disconnection. It is within the confines of this fear that stereotypes and misconceptions flourish, inhibiting the natural flow of sexual energy and curiosity.

Sometimes, these barriers extend into the realm of anxiety and stress. The pressures of modern life, coupled with personal insecurities, manifest as anxiety that spills over into our sexual lives. This anxiety could stem from performance expectations or apprehension about intimacy, both of which can stifle sexual enjoyment and impede emotional connection.

Another key barrier is the presence of unresolved trauma, often lurking underneath the surface. Traumatic experiences, particularly those related to sexual history, profoundly influence sexual identity and functioning. They can create protective walls that hinder intimate relationships, making it difficult to build trust or engage in fulfilling sexual interactions.

Negative self-image and poor body confidence represent additional hurdles on the path to healthy sexual expression. In a world bombarded by images of 'ideal' beauty, individuals may find themselves trapped in cycles of self-criticism. This fixation on perceived imperfections can diminish sexual confidence, curbing one's ability to feel desirable or engage freely in intimate moments.

These barriers, however, are not insurmountable. Recognising and confronting them marks the first step towards liberation and healing. It involves a process akin to peeling back layers of an onion, each one uncovering earlier and deeper sources of discomfort. This journey requires patience, introspection, and often, external support.

Therapeutic interventions can be particularly effective in navigating these psychological landscapes. Engaging with a skilled therapist provides a safe space to explore and dismantle the narratives that perpetuate these barriers. Therapeutic modalities such as cognitive-behavioural therapy, mindfulness-based approaches, and somatic experiencing offer frameworks to reinterpret and integrate past experiences positively.

Moreover, cultivating a practice of mindfulness can help in recognising and altering thought patterns that contribute to these barriers. Mindfulness encourages presence in the moment, helping individuals to tune into their bodies and emotions without judgement. This practice can foster a deeper understanding of personal needs and desires, creating a healthier relationship with one's sexual self.

Building open lines of communication with partners also plays a crucial role in overcoming psychological barriers. Discussing fears, insecurities, and desires can break down the walls that isolate individuals within their thoughts. Such conversations require vulnerability and courage but pave the way for increased intimacy and mutual understanding.

Education is another tool in dismantling psychological barriers. Being informed about sexual health and rights can empower individuals to challenge misconceptions and set healthy boundaries. Access to comprehensive and diverse sexual education can illuminate paths towards acceptance and freedom, reducing the impact of societal and internalised stigmas.

Lastly, fostering a supportive community can significantly ease the journey towards overcoming psychological barriers. Engaging with others who resonate with similar experiences can provide validation and encouragement. Communities can be a source of strength and insight, helping individuals to feel less isolated in their challenges and more inspired to embrace their sexual truth.

While psychological barriers may feel daunting, they offer fertile ground for personal growth and transformation. Each step taken to challenge these barriers builds resilience, self-awareness, and a deeper connection to one's desires. By addressing these obstacles, individuals open themselves to more profound and fulfilling sexual expression, integral to their overall well-being.

Embarking on this journey calls for compassion towards oneself and the courage to face what lies beneath the surface. It is through this exploration that we can transcend limitations and allow our sexual expression to become a source of joy, healing, and empowerment.

The Role of Mindfulness in Sexual Health

The interplay between mindfulness and sexual health represents an intriguing frontier in the journey toward holistic well-being. In the midst of our chaotic lives, the ability to anchor oneself in the present moment can profoundly transform experiences, particularly those as intimate and personal as sexual encounters. Mindfulness, at its core, involves an intentional focus on the here and now, free from judgment or distraction. This mindfulness, when applied to sexual health, unlocks a pathway to a more profound and satisfying sexual expression.

Mindful sexual practice often begins with self-awareness. By tuning into one's own body, emotions, and sensations, individuals can gain a deeper understanding of their personal desires and boundaries. This self-awareness acts as a bridge to more authentic sexual expression, allowing one to communicate these insights to a partner. It's not merely about enhancing sensory experiences; it's about recognising and honouring one's inner landscape.

Consider the act of deep breathing—a fundamental mindfulness technique. During moments of intimacy, deep breathing can help centre the mind, reducing anxiety and enhancing physiological responses. As stress diminishes, so too do the barriers that often impede sexual desire and satisfaction. Breathing becomes a tool for connection, grounding couples in shared presence and intention.

Moreover, mindfulness encourages a mindset shift—from goal-oriented outcomes to an appreciation of the journey itself. Sexual experiences often carry societal pressures of performance and expectation. By focusing on the present, individuals can become more attuned to the subtleties of pleasure, exploring texture, temperature, and movement without the weight of expectation. This openness fosters a richer understanding of personal and partnered experiences, enhancing both self-love and mutual respect.

Focusing on mindful awareness also cultivates a profound sense of empathy and connection with sexual partners. Relationships often falter when communication breaks down, but mindfulness requires active listening and presence. This attentiveness translates to more meaningful interactions, where individuals fully engage with their partners' needs and responses. By being present, one validates their partner's experiences, nurturing a space where vulnerability and trust can flourish.

Yet, the journey toward mindfulness in sexual health isn't without its challenges. It requires practice and patience, especially in a world that often prioritises haste over reflection. The key lies in consistent, intentional practice. Consider integrating short mindfulness sessions into daily routines, gradually extending these practices into intimate settings. As with any skill, proficiency develops over time, rewarding individuals with heightened intimacy and satisfaction.

Additionally, mindful sexual health promotes the dismantling of harmful scripts and narratives surrounding sexuality. When individuals become more present, they can challenge preconceived notions ingrained by past experiences and societal norms. This allows for a more personal and liberated form of sexual expression, unencumbered by shame or comparison. Acceptance and self-compassion become the cornerstones of sexual experiences.

Let's not forget the profound mental health benefits that emerge from this mindful approach. Sexual health and mental health are inherently interconnected, each influencing the other's trajectory. Mindfulness acts as a stabilising force, mitigating anxiety and depression's adverse effects on sexual expression. It offers a sanctuary from the relentless busyness of life, allowing sexual well-being to flourish unhindered.

Enhancing sexual health through mindfulness also invites a broader exploration of erotic energy, not as something to be controlled, but as a vibrant life force to be embraced. By leaning into awareness, individuals can harness this energy for personal empowerment and healing, expanding their understanding of sensuality and embodiment.

In empowering individuals to own their sexual journeys, mindfulness nurtures a tapestry of experiences that extend beyond the bedroom. It enhances confidence in everyday life, encouraging individuals to reflect on what truly brings joy and fulfilment. Whether through solo practice or shared experiences, the mindful path carves out spaces for creativity, exploration, and growth.

The practical application of mindfulness in sexual health unveils myriad opportunities for both individuals and couples seeking deeper connections. Workshops, retreats, and therapy programs often offer guided mindfulness practices tailored specifically to enhance sexual well-being. By exploring these avenues, individuals and partners can embark on collective paths towards rejuvenated intimacy and connection.

By integrating mindfulness into sexual experiences, individuals remind themselves that sexual health is neither isolated nor secondary to overall well-being; rather, it is deeply intertwined with mental, emotional, and physical health. This comprehensive approach emphasises that true sexual empowerment emerges when mindfulness becomes a staple, not an exception, in one's daily life.

As we conclude this exploration into the role of mindfulness in sexual health, it becomes clear that the practice is far more than a fleeting trend. It is a transformative process that invites individuals to fully engage with themselves and their partners, fostering an environment where intimacy and connection thrive. One step at a time, mindfulness can reshape the narrative of sexual health, leading to a fulfilling and balanced life.

Chapter 6:
Social Influences on Sexual Well-being

The social landscape profoundly shapes our sexual well-being, weaving complex patterns through our lives that can either nurture or hinder our sexual health. From cultural norms that subtly dictate what's considered "acceptable" to societal expectations that often weigh heavily on individuals, these influences are omnipresent and powerful. At the heart of this dynamic lies the interplay between personal relationships and collective beliefs. Our interactions with partners, friends, and even the media can either bolster a healthy sense of sexual self or lead to internalised negativity and confusion. But embracing this awareness is empowering—by recognising and critically analysing these social cues, one can navigate relationships with a deeper understanding and more resilience. The journey towards sexual well-being involves not just an exploration of our inner desires but also a mindful interrogation of the social currents around us, allowing us to forge connections that are genuine and fulfilling.

Cultural Norms and Their Impact

The tapestry of human sexuality is intricately woven with cultural threads, which shape our perceptions, attitudes, and behaviours regarding sexual well-being. Cultural norms, those unwritten rules of conduct that pervade society, have a profound influence on how we understand and engage with our sexual selves. It's important to recognise that these norms are neither fixed nor universal; they vary significantly across different societies and periods. Understanding their role and impact on sexual well-being can lead to a more fulfilling and liberated experience of sexuality.

Cultural norms often dictate the acceptable parameters of sexual behaviour, influencing everything from the expression of desire to the structure of intimate relationships. For instance, in some cultures, premarital sex might be viewed with disfavour, while in others, it is considered a natural progression of romantic involvement. The way we experience guilt, shame, or pride related to our sexual choices can be deeply rooted in these societal expectations. In cultures where open discussion of sex is taboo, individuals may struggle to seek information and support, negatively impacting their sexual health.

Historical contexts also play a significant role in shaping cultural norms. For example, Victorian-era attitudes towards sex, steeped in restraint and propriety, continue to echo in modern societies, affecting contemporary views on modesty and virginity. These historical legacies can often lead to the perpetuation of stereotypes and myths about sexuality, ultimately inhibiting personal growth and sexual freedom.

Moreover, cultural norms influence gender roles, which in turn affect sexual dynamics and expectations. Traditional gender roles, often characterised by distinct behavioural expectations for men and women, can limit the expression of authentic desire. In some contexts, men might feel pressured to exhibit hyper-masculinity, equating sexual conquest with success, while women might encounter pressure to appear modest or chaste. Such roles can lead to misunderstandings and dissatisfaction within relationships, restricting individuals from exploring their true sexual identities.

Despite potentially restrictive aspects, cultural norms can also provide a framework for connecting with others and constructing identities. They can foster community cohesion, giving people a sense of belonging and shared understanding. Positive cultural norms, such as those promoting mutual respect and consent, can enhance sexual wellbeing by creating environments where individuals feel safe and valued. Encouraging open dialogue about sexual health can break down barriers and empower people to make informed choices.

Globalisation and the exchange of cultural ideas through media and travel have led to the cross-pollination of sexual norms. Exposure to diverse cultural perspectives can challenge conventional norms and encourage individuals to redefine their boundaries and expectations. This blending of cultural influences offers the opportunity for more flexible, inclusive views of sexuality, fostering a landscape where diverse expressions and identities are celebrated rather than suppressed.

As we navigate the myriad influences of cultural norms on sexual well-being, it becomes crucial to cultivate an awareness of their impact on personal and collective levels. Breaking free of limiting beliefs requires introspection and often courage, to challenge and perhaps alter ingrained societal scripts. Embracing the potential for change does not mean discarding tradition completely, but rather recognising which moments from tradition serve our collective well-being and which serve only to constrain.

Encouraging conversations around sexuality, both personal and public, can dismantle harmful stereotypes and illuminate paths towards greater sexual autonomy. By advocating for open, honest discourse about sex, societies can uplift individuals, empower relationships, and transform cultural landscapes into nurturing spaces for sexual expression. Additionally, sex education that is inclusive and honest is paramount in fostering sexual well-being across all ages, providing the tools needed for understanding and respecting diversity in sexual expression.

Ultimately, understanding the intersection of cultural norms and sexual well-being is an ongoing journey. It's about recognising the influence these norms have had and continue to have on our lives, and working proactively to ensure they support more liberated and healthy expressions of sexuality. This awareness empowers individuals to forge paths that align with their authentic selves, leading to richer, healthier relationships with themselves and others.

Navigating Relationships and Expectations

In the realm of sexual well-being, the intricate dance between relationships and societal expectations often dictates how we perceive and experience intimacy. At its core, navigating relationships involves understanding the complex interplay between personal desires and external pressures. These pressures can stem from cultural norms, family influences, or even our own constructed ideals about what a relationship should look like.

Everyone brings their own set of expectations into a relationship, and these expectations are often shaped long before we even realise. From fairy tales to modern media portrayals, we're bombarded with often unrealistic ideals of romance and partnership. These narratives can set up false benchmarks, leading to dissatisfaction when reality inevitably differs from the scripted plotlines. Recognising that these portrayals might not serve us is the first step towards fostering a healthier connection.

Communication is the cornerstone for balancing personal needs with partner expectations. It's important to have open discussions about desires, boundaries, and mutual aspirations. The ability to convey what one wants and needs—without judgement or fear—builds trust. Trust, in turn, reinforces the relationship's foundation, allowing for more meaningful and satisfying sexual interactions. It's not just about being heard; it's about truly listening and responding to a partner's needs.

The art of compromise, while crucial, shouldn't mean diluting one's self wholly to accommodate another. Healthy relationships thrive on a balance—where both parties have room to express their individuality and growth without feeling tethered by obligation. This balance fosters a sense of security and belonging, both of which are essential for a fulfilling sexual relationship.

Moreover, understanding the macro-elements that influence our relationships is equally important. The societal lens through which relationships are viewed can exert considerable pressure. For example, traditional roles can sometimes stifle authentic expression, pushing individuals into roles that don't align with their true selves. Challenging these norms can be liberating, allowing for more authentic connections that are based on mutual respect and understanding.

There's also the aspect of managing expectations that are self-imposed. Often, these expectations are built on internalised beliefs about perfection and inadequacy, which can colour our interactions with others. By understanding the origins of these beliefs, individuals can begin to dismantle them, paving the way for more genuine expressions of affection and desire.

The journey towards sexual well-being within a relationship isn't without its trials. Navigating expectations, both external and internal, requires patience and empathy. It's important to remember that no relationship is devoid of challenges, but it's how these challenges are addressed that determines the overall health of the partnership. Challenges offer opportunities to learn and adapt, not just to compromise or concede.

Furthermore, embracing change can be a powerful approach to handling expectations. As relationships evolve, so too can the dynamics within them. What might have worked well at the beginning may need revisiting later. Open channels of dialogue about these shifts can prevent misunderstandings and resentment. Change doesn't necessarily signal the end; often, it's an invitation to grow together.

In touching on relationships and expectations, self-awareness cannot be understated. Knowing one's own desires, boundaries, and fears is crucial. This self-awareness not only enriches personal growth but also enhances the relational dynamic. By being in tune with oneself, the ability to recognise the same in others expands, leading to deeper and more meaningful connections.

Ultimately, navigating relationships and expectations is about pursuing joy and fulfilment, not just settling for an idealised notion of what should be. When relationships are crafted with intention and care, they become supportive environments where sexual well-being can flourish naturally. Instead of adhering to rigid frameworks, seek to establish a shared vision that evolves as the relationship does. This flexibility creates a fertile ground for both personal and shared growth.

Navigating these terrains with genuine curiosity and open-mindedness can lead to profound transformations. In embracing the fluidity of expectations, individuals and couples can find liberation and satisfaction that ripple through every aspect of their lives, deepening their overall sense of well-being.

Chapter 7:
Nutrition and Sexual Vitality

Nourishment plays a profound role in the dance of sexual vitality, acting as a foundation upon which desire flourishes. Our bodies are intricate mechanisms that respond keenly to what we consume, meaning that the food we ingest isn't just fuel for daily tasks, but also a catalyst for passion and intimacy. Foods rich in essential nutrients, like zinc and omega-3 fatty acids, help bolster hormone levels and blood circulation, both of which are crucial for fostering a healthy libido. Vibrant fruits, vegetables, and whole grains can invigorate not just our physical health but also our desire, promoting a natural sense of vitality. Understanding the connection between diet and libido empowers us to make conscious choices that enhance both our sexual health and overall well-being, helping us to lead a life that's not only balanced but also joyously fulfilling.

Foods that Fuel Desire

When it comes to bolstering one's sexual vitality, nutrition plays a crucial role. Just like how the body demands fuel to function effectively, our sexual health requires specific nutrients to thrive. There's a fascinating dance between what we consume and how we feel, and amidst this choreography, certain foods emerge as stars, known for their ability to ignite desire and boost sexual energy.

Nature has endowed us with an array of aphrodisiacs, renowned not for their mystical properties but for their undeniable connection to increased libido and energy. Take, for example, the humble oyster. Rich in zinc, a mineral imperative for testosterone production, oysters have long been hailed for their ability to boost sexual desire. The role of testosterone in both men and women is pivotal for maintaining sexual drive, and even small enhancements in this hormone can lead to significant upticks in desire.

Then there's chocolate, the silky confection that has captured the hearts (and senses) of many. But chocolate is more than just a sweet treat. Packed with phenylethylamine and serotonin, it stimulates pleasure centres in the brain, creating a feeling of euphoria similar to that of falling in love. Dark chocolate, in particular, is rich in antioxidants, promoting better blood flow and thus enhancing sexual function.

While some foods stimulate the senses, others work quietly behind the scenes, ensuring our hormonal balance is spot-on. Nuts and seeds, particularly almonds and sunflower seeds, are rich in healthy fats and vitamin E. These nutrients are essential for hormone production and overall sexual health. They help maintain the integrity of cell membranes, and ensuring robust cellular function is critical for hormonal activities, including sex hormone synthesis.

Let's not overlook the sultry chili pepper, with its fiery kick. Capsaicin, the compound that gives chili peppers their heat, stimulates endorphins and enhances blood circulation – both of which are vital for sexual arousal and desire. A dash of spicy food can raise heartbeats, mirroring the physiological effects of sexual excitement.

Garlic might not be the first food that comes to mind when considering romance, owing to its pungent aroma. Yet, it contains allicin, which increases blood flow, a critical factor in increased libido. Regular consumption can make a significant difference in sexual health, particularly in boosting endurance.

In the world of fruits, bananas stand out not only for their suggestive appearance but for their wealth of B vitamins and potassium. These nutrients enhance the body's capacity to produce sex hormones, promoting an increased sexual drive and energy level. Similarly, figs and avocados have been historically celebrated for their fertility-boosting properties, tied to their abundance of vitamins, minerals, and healthy fats.

Leafy greens like spinach and kale are powerhouses of magnesium, a mineral that decreases inflammation and improves blood flow. Better blood circulation means more efficient delivery of nutrients and oxygen throughout the body, including to the sexual organs, enhancing performance and pleasure.

Hydration, too, plays a pivotal role in maintaining sexual health. A glass of watermelon juice can do wonders; packed with citrulline, this fruit helps relax blood vessels and improve circulation, almost acting as a natural Viagra. In a similar vein, beetroots are potent in nitrates that expand blood vessels, ensuring that pleasure is not only felt but sustained.

While these foods can set the stage for heightened desire and improved sexual function, it's essential to see them as part of a holistic approach to nutrition. A balanced diet rich in fruits, vegetables, lean proteins, and whole grains supports overall health, which is intimately tied to sexual vitality. Moreover, it's crucial to be mindful of reducing processed foods high in sugars and unhealthy fats, as they can have the opposite effect, impeding sexual health by causing sluggishness, poor circulation, and hormonal imbalances.

Incorporating these foods into one's diet doesn't mean drastic changes or bland meals. Think of a vibrant salad loaded with leafy greens, sprinkled with seeds and nuts, adorned with slices of avocado. Or picture a dish drizzled with chilli-infused olive oil, accompanied by a side of roasted beetroots. There's not only room for indulgence and enjoyment but a reminder that pleasure starts with the conscious choice of what we put into our bodies.

Equally important is the context in which we consume these foods. Sharing meals with a partner or creating an ambiance of warmth and connection can elevate the experience altogether. Dining becomes more than mere sustenance; it transforms into a ritual that binds us closer to our desires and to each other.

Food, in its essence, is deeply intertwined with the art of seduction and the celebration of life and love. By choosing wisely and dining mindfully, we can enhance not only the flavours on our plate but the depth and richness of our intimate lives.

In nurturing our bodies with these foods that fuel desire, we're also embracing a lifestyle that aligns with optimal sexual health. The journey towards enhanced sexual vitality doesn't begin with a magic pill but rather with conscious, everyday choices that honour the intricate connection between nourishment and desire. So, as we savour each bite, let us be reminded of the powerful potential within us to cultivate a sexually vibrant and fulfilling life.

The Connection Between Diet and Libido

The intimate link between what we eat and our sexual vitality is a topic that intertwines the very essence of our daily choices with the primal drive of libido. In a world where instant gratification often overshadows the subtle art of nurturing the body, understanding the dynamic connection between diet and sexual desire is more important than ever. A balanced and thoughtful approach to nutrition can enhance our sexual well-being, making it an integral component of our overall health.

At its core, libido—or sexual desire—is influenced by a delicate balance of hormones and neurotransmitters. These chemical messengers in the body are, in turn, profoundly affected by the nutrients we consume. For instance, omega-3 fatty acids, found abundantly in oily fish like salmon or sardines, play a significant role in maintaining optimal hormone levels. They assist in the production of dopamine, a neurotransmitter that promotes pleasure and desire.

Moreover, the amino acid arginine, which is prevalent in foods like nuts, seeds, and certain meats, contributes to the production of nitric oxide. This compound is essential for vasodilation, a process that increases blood flow to all body parts, including the genitals, enhancing arousal and sensation. So, by including such nutrient-rich foods in our diet, we actively participate in sustaining both our physical and sexual vitality.

Is there any truth to the notion of aphrodisiacs, those legendary substances purported to spark desire? While some claims are steeped in myth, certain foods do have particular compounds that can have a suggestive effect on desire. Take chocolate, for instance. It's often called an aphrodisiac due to the presence of phenylethylamine (PEA), a compound that can create a feeling of excitement and wellbeing. Of course, moderation is key, and it's not the chocolate that holds the magic but the chemical reaction it sparks within us.

Zinc also plays a vital role in the realm of diet and sexual health. This mineral is crucial in testosterone production, which is linked to libido in both men and women. Oysters are famously high in zinc, hence their reputation for enhancing desire. But zinc can also be sourced from plant-based foods like seeds, nuts, and whole grains, offering plenty of options to suit various dietary preferences.

Interestingly, the interplay between diet and libido emphasises the importance of gut health. A balanced gut microbiome supports nutrient absorption and optimal hormone production. Fermented foods such as yogurt, kimchi, and sauerkraut are excellent for promoting a healthy balance of gut bacteria. This connection underlines that dietary choices impact not just immediate bodily functions but deeper systemic health, which ultimately influences our capacity to experience desire and pleasure.

Aside from individual nutrients, the overall patterns of eating significantly impact sexual health. Both the Mediterranean and DASH diets, known for their heart-healthy benefits, have also been linked to enhanced sexual function. These diets promote a high intake of fruits, vegetables, whole grains, and healthy fats, which support cardiovascular health and, consequently, sexual function.

The effects of poor dietary choices on libido should not be overlooked. Excessive consumption of processed foods high in sugar and unhealthy fats may contribute to hormonal imbalances and reduced sexual desire. Such foods can lead to inflammation and insulin resistance, further compromising vascular health and the body's ability to manage stress, which in turn can dampen sexual desire.

Alcohol also plays a double-edged role. In moderation, it might lower inhibitions and create a more relaxed atmosphere conducive to intimacy. However, excessive consumption can have severe implications, including decreased sexual performance and testosterone production. Restraint and mindfulness in consumption are critical to preserving both health and libido.

Aside from what we eat, when we eat can also shape our sexual wellness. Maintaining regular meal times helps stabilise blood sugar levels and prevent energy crashes, which can negatively affect mood and libido. Eating together with a partner can offer emotional connectivity and acts as an intimate practice in itself, enhancing the overall experience of shared meals.

Ultimately, each individual's nutritional journey is unique, and finding a diet that aligns with one's personal health needs and goals is crucial. Listening to the body, paying attention to how different foods affect energy levels, mood, and desire, allows us to make informed choices that support both our physical and sexual health.

Integrating these insights into daily life doesn't mean overhauling one's diet overnight. Making gradual changes, experimenting with nutrient-rich recipes, and enjoying the discovery of how these adjustments impact overall wellbeing can transform the relationship with food into a source of empowerment.

Thus, as we conclude this exploration of diet and libido, it is paramount to remember that nurturing our bodies with intention and care is not merely about sustenance. It is about celebrating our primal urges and recognising the potential for pleasure in everyday choices. Embracing this connection can lead to a more fulfilled, invigorated life where nutrition and sexual vitality move in harmony.

Chapter 8:
Physical Fitness and Sexual Health

In the journey towards holistic well-being, the synergy between physical fitness and sexual health emerges as a transformative force. Our bodies, vibrant and dynamic, thrive on movement, and regular exercise becomes a catalyst for enhancing sexual well-being. It is not just about cultivating strength and endurance but fostering a deeper connection with oneself. By engaging in activities that elevate the heart rate and invigorate the senses, individuals can experience improved circulation, heightened arousal, and a boost in confidence—all crucial elements for a fulfilling sex life. Furthermore, practices like yoga, with its focus on breath and alignment, offer profound benefits by balancing energy and increasing body awareness, thus enriching sexual desire. Embracing physical movement not only rejuvenates the body but also liberates the mind, allowing for an empowered, unapologetic expression of one's sexuality. This chapter beckons you to explore how intentionally nurturing your physical fitness can lead to a more harmonious and satisfying sexual life, paving the way for a balanced and enriched existence.

Exercise for Enhancing Sexual Well-being

An invigorating exercise routine can be a cornerstone for a fulfilled sexual life, offering both physical and emotional benefits that transcend mere physicality. Enhanced circulation, increased endorphins, and reduced stress levels, all contribute to a healthy libido.

Physical activity isn't just about how your body looks; it's about how your body feels and performs in all aspects of life, including the intimate ones.

Vigorous exercise such as running, swimming, or even a spirited cycle through the countryside has profound effects on your sexual well-being. These activities boost cardiovascular health, which is crucial for stamina and endurance—qualities that directly impact sexual performance. Increased blood flow, resulting from regular cardiovascular exercise, supports erectile function in men and heightened arousal in women. Moreover, the release of endorphins acts as a natural stress reliever, creating a mental space where desire can flourish.

Strength training, often considered the purview of bodybuilders and elite athletes, brings sculptural benefits to the body. However, it also profoundly impacts sexual well-being. By engaging in strength exercises, you improve your muscle tone, which can enhance sexual confidence. Feeling strong and capable in your own skin fosters a positive body image, encouraging more adventurous and pleasurable sexual experiences. Moreover, strong muscles contribute to better control and endurance during sex, facilitating prolonged pleasure.

Don't underestimate the power of flexibility and balance exercises such as Pilates or Tai Chi. Flexibility enhances the range of motion, allowing couples to experiment and enjoy various positions without discomfort. Tai Chi, often praised for its meditative movements, builds a strong core and improves balance, elements that guide you toward more fulfilling encounters. The practice brings tranquility and focus, clearing away mental distractions that can impede intimacy.

Interestingly, high-intensity interval training (HIIT) can also offer unique benefits for sexual health. The short, intense bursts of exercise followed by short recovery periods mimic the variability seen in sexual activity. It teaches the body to cope with rapid changes in intensity and exertion, mirroring the dynamics of an engaging sexual experience. HIIT workouts are efficient, time-saving, and can lead to improved cardiovascular fitness, which is vital for sustained sexual energy and stamina.

The connection between regular exercise and improved mood is well-documented and should not be overlooked. Activities that you genuinely enjoy, like dancing, can release feel-good hormones and decrease anxiety, fostering a positive environment for sexual desire. Dancing, with its rhythm and flow, is not only a fun way to stay fit but it enhances body awareness and coordination, both of which can contribute to more synchronized and satisfying sexual experiences.

Group sports or team-based physical activities also offer a distinctive benefit to sexual well-being. The camaraderie and social interactions present opportunities for building relationships and boosting self-esteem. The confidence gained through teamwork and achieving common goals can transfer to personal relationships, encouraging a more open and connected sexual experience with your partner.

Consider the role of mental focus in physical fitness; exercises like rock climbing or martial arts demand concentration and attention, creating a mindfulness that can translate into your sex life. This level of focus can help in being fully present during intimate encounters, heightening the overall experience for both partners. When you learn to concentrate your energy and attention during physical activities, it enhances your ability to connect deeply during sexual activity.

Incorporating a variety of exercises into your routine not only benefits your physical health but also addresses different aspects of sexual well-being. Overcoming sexual challenges with a multi-faceted fitness approach keeps you motivated and engaged, significantly enhancing your sexual vitality.

Explore activities that might be new to you. The thrill of trying something different, like aerial yoga or paddleboarding, can reignite passion and excitement, qualities essential for vibrant sexual health. Engaging in such diverse exercises can stimulate both your physical and mental faculties, reminding you of the joy to be found in exploration and adaptation.

Exercise, essentially, isn't just about discipline and routine; it's about discovery. Discover what feels good, what empowers you, and what rekindles your energy. Recognising and supporting each aspect of your health through physical fitness can lead you to a place where your sexual well-being is bolstered, ensuring it becomes a priority in your journey towards overall well-being.

The most essential takeaway is to choose exercises that complement your lifestyle and speak to your interests. When exercise is enjoyable rather than obligatory, it transforms into a sustainable practice. The link between regular physical activity and enhanced sexual health should be embraced as an opportunity to grow, not as a chore. This integration of physical fitness into your life can create a ripple effect, enhancing not just your sexual well-being, but enriching every area of your life.

Yoga and Its Benefits for Desire

In the intricate tapestry of physical fitness and sexual health, yoga emerges as a profound practice that extends beyond the boundaries of the mat. It seamlessly integrates breath, movement, and mindfulness, creating a holistic approach to enhancing sexual desire. Yoga is not merely an exercise; it's a transformative practice that fosters a deeper connection with oneself. Through its diverse postures and meditative elements, yoga can significantly influence sexual vitality—leading to an enriched and balanced life.

At its core, yoga encourages an awareness of one's body, promoting a sense of presence that is crucial for sexual health. This awareness is cultivated through poses that open the hips and pelvis, regions intrinsically connected to sexual energy and desire. When these areas are tense or blocked, desire can be inhibited. By practising yoga postures such as the pigeon pose or the bound angle pose, one can release physical tension and emotional blockages, thus facilitating a more liberated expression of desire.

Beyond the physical release, yoga is also a journey into your own psyche, unearthing the layers that often conceal true desires. Regular practice helps break down barriers erected by stress, anxiety, and negative self-perceptions. By integrating body and mind, yoga practitioners often find themselves more open to exploration and self-acceptance. This openness is a critical component of a healthy sexual life, as it encourages authenticity and confidence in personal and intimate settings.

One cannot overstate the significance of breathwork within yoga practice and its impact on sexual health. Pranayama, the practice of controlled breathing, is vital. It aids in the reduction of cortisol levels, the hormone associated with stress, which can be a major deterrent to sexual desire. Deep, intentional breaths bring focus, enhance relaxation, and increase circulation, all of which are pivotal to healthy sexual function. As the breath deepens, so does one's capacity for pleasure, as increased oxygen flow invigorates the body and cultivates a heightened sense of awareness.

Yoga's influence extends to mental health, an essential element of cultivating and maintaining desire. The meditative aspects of yoga can lead to a decreased perception of stress and a notable rise in happiness and satisfaction. These mental states are directly correlated with a positive sexual outlook. When one feels mentally at ease, the mind becomes a playground for curiosity and imagination, both vital for sustaining desire.

Furthermore, yoga contributes to better hormonal balance, which is crucial for sexual health. Certain yoga poses stimulate the endocrine system by nurturing glands like the thyroid and adrenal glands, which regulate hormones responsible for sexual desire. A balanced endocrine system can lead to a natural increase in libido, providing a more spontaneous and enriched sexual experience.

The practice of yoga fosters an intimate connection, not only within oneself but also with one's partner. Partner yoga, in particular, opens avenues for physical and emotional bonding. It requires communication, trust, and a shared presence, enhancing intimacy outside the realms of physical intercourse. By moving in harmony, partners may discover new dimensions of their relationship, reinforcing their togetherness and shared desires.

Emotionally, yoga cultivates resilience. It teaches acceptance and patience—qualities that spill over into the sexual aspects of one's life. Learning to accept one's imperfections and those of others can release overwhelming pressures of sexual performance or expectations. As a result, desire becomes a natural expression, comfortably free from constraints.

Moreover, yoga can amplify body positivity. In the process of mastering poses and flows, practitioners often find themselves gaining a new appreciation for their bodies. This self-love leads to an increase in confidence and self-esteem, creating a fertile ground for sexual desire to thrive. The more comfortable one is in their skin, the more likely they are to enjoy and engage in fulfilling sexual experiences.

Socially, the community aspect of yoga shouldn't be overlooked. Sharing a collective goal with fellow practitioners can provide a sense of belonging and support. This communal experience can lead to increased emotional well-being, which directly impacts how one perceives and experiences desire. The inspiration and motivation drawn from a community can transform personal practice into a shared celebration of vitality and passion.

Ultimately, integrating yoga into one's lifestyle forms a synergistic relationship between physical fitness and sexual health. It offers tools to channel both physical and emotional states into a positive cycle of well-being. By fostering mindfulness, resilience, and self-awareness, yoga becomes a cornerstone for enhancing desire—a thread woven intricately into the fabric of life. In this continuous journey of personal growth, yoga not only enriches physical health but also deepens and empowers interpersonal connections, enabling individuals to embrace their sexuality with confidence and joy.

Chapter 9:
Harnessing Erotic Energy for Health

In the realm of holistic well-being, erotic energy emerges as a powerful force that can enrich both our physical health and emotional resilience. When harnessed with intention, this potent energy not only enhances intimacy but also fosters a deeper connection to oneself and others. Techniques for cultivating sexual energy, such as breathwork and mindful movement, open the gateways to vibrant wellness. These practices encourage the body to channel erotic energy constructively, promoting healing and a sense of wholeness. The healing power of eroticism isn't just a metaphor; it's a tangible vitality that elevates our mood, sharpens our creativity, and fortifies our spirit. As we embrace our erotic potential, we nurture not just our sexual health, but our entire being, weaving a tapestry of wellness that's as fulfilling as it is transformative.

Techniques for Cultivating Sexual Energy

Understanding and harnessing sexual energy is a journey toward a more vibrant and fulfilling life. It's about tapping into a wellspring of vitality that not only enhances intimate relationships but also feeds into your overall well-being. Like any form of energy, sexual energy can be cultivated, channelled, and transformed. Diverse traditions and modern practices offer avenues to explore this potency within us.

One of the foundational steps in cultivating sexual energy is awareness. This awareness is not merely a cognitive exercise; it invites you to pay close attention to the sensations in your body, the rhythms of your breath, and the ebb and flow of desire. Engaging in mindful breathing exercises can serve as a gateway to becoming attuned to these sexual energies. With each inhale, imagine drawing in life-giving energy, and with each exhale, release tension and negativity. This simple practice can prepare your body and mind for deeper exploration of sexual energy.

Another powerful technique is movement, especially meditative movement. Practices like Tai Chi, Qigong, and even certain forms of dance can harmonise your body's energy. These forms of movement emphasize fluidity and connection, encouraging a conscious engagement with the body that enhances sensitivity to sexual energy. As you move, focus on the energy pathways within your body, and allow them to become channels through which sexual vitality can freely flow.

For many, the ancient art of Tantra offers profound insights into the cultivation of sexual energy. Far from being merely sexual in nature, Tantric practices teach a way of life that embraces sexuality as a sacred force. Tantra encourages the merging of physical and spiritual energies, fostering a state of heightened awareness and greater connectivity between partners. Techniques may include meditative practices, breathwork, and rituals that emphasise the interconnectedness of all aspects of life.

It's important to mention the role of the pelvic floor in nurturing sexual energy. Exercises aimed at strengthening these muscles, commonly referred to as Kegel exercises, can enhance sexual pleasure and potency for all genders. By increasing control and awareness of these muscles, individuals often report a marked improvement in their sexual experiences and energy levels.

The mind-body connection is also crucial in managing and directing sexual energy. Visualisation techniques can be instrumental in this regard. Start by closing your eyes and envisioning your sexual energy as a warm, glowing light residing at your core. With each breath, see this light expanding, filling your entire being with warmth and vitality. This exercise can amplify your awareness of sexual energy and contribute to a greater sense of empowerment.

Additionally, cultivating sexual energy involves recognizing and respecting personal boundaries. Emotional safety is paramount, as it creates a nurturing environment for energy to flourish. Engaging in open and honest communication with partners can lay the groundwork for this safety. Express your needs, desires, and limits clearly, fostering a relationship built on trust and mutual exploration.

Nourishment is another facet to consider. What you consume, both physically and emotionally, impacts your sexual vitality. Incorporating foods known to enhance libido and energy, such as avocados, nuts, and dark chocolate, can have a positive effect. Equally important is feeding the mind with positive affirmations and constructive thoughts about sexuality and self-worth.

Recharging your sexual energy also means taking time for solitude and reflection. In a world often filled with noise and distraction, finding quiet moments can be challenging yet rewarding. Use this time to journal, meditate, or simply be. These reflective practices allow for the internalisation of sexual energy, enabling it to rejuvenate rather than deplete you.

Ultimately, the goal is not to control or suppress sexual energy but to embrace it as an integral component of your life. Celebrating this energy infuses your everyday with creativity, joy, and passion, echoing into every aspect of your existence. By integrating these techniques, you start to weave a rich tapestry where sexual energy is cherished, respected, and optimally utilised.

Remember, cultivating sexual energy is deeply personal, and what works for one individual might differ for another. It requires patience, openness, and a willingness to explore diverse approaches. As with any aspect of self-discovery, the journey is as significant as the destination. Each exploration brings you closer to understanding your true self, ultimately leading to a more harmonious connection with those around you and a greater sense of personal enlightenment.

The Healing Power of Eroticism

Eroticism is more than just a fleeting moment of passion. It is a profound force that holds the potential to heal, transform, and invigorate our lives. At its core, eroticism is about the sensual and the emotional, weaving together threads of intimacy, excitement, and curiosity into a tapestry that enriches our health and well-being. This healing power emerges when we allow ourselves to fully engage with our erotic selves, shedding societal taboos and embracing our natural desires.

For many, eroticism carries a heavy burden of misconceptions, often seen solely through the lens of physical acts or reduced to mere carnal pleasures. However, at its essence, it represents a deep-seated connection to one's sense of identity and vitality. To harness this energy for health, it's critical to explore eroticism as a holistic experience, transcending the physical and delving into emotional and spiritual realms. The sensual awareness that eroticism fosters can act as a remedy to the stresses of everyday life, offering a sanctuary wherein one can safely explore and heal.

Throughout history, societies have recognised the healing power inherent in erotic energy. Ancient cultures often celebrated sexuality as a vital force of nature, integrating sexual rites and practices into their spiritual and healing traditions. These perspectives are not just relics of the past; they hint at an understanding that aligns physical pleasure with emotional and spiritual well-being. By reclaiming these notions, we can appreciate how eroticism, in all its complexities, nurtures us holistically.

Emotionally, the embrace of erotic energy can bridge gaps created by life's stresses. In relationships, allowing eroticism to flourish can reignite passion and improve communication. When both partners are attuned to one another's desires, the intimate bond strengthens, acting as a buffer against the negative impacts of daily pressures. This energy encourages vulnerability, allowing individuals to express their true selves, creating an emotional intimacy that is both healing and affirming.

Moreover, engaging with one's erotic self can significantly impact mental health. When we acknowledge and honour our desires, we give ourselves permission to exist authentically, free from the shackles of shame and guilt that often accompany sexual expression in modern society. This liberation supports mental resilience, reducing stress and anxiety, and promoting a positive outlook towards life. Embracing eroticism can be a powerful form of self-affirmation, encouraging a narrative where one feels worthy of pleasure and love.

On a physical level, the benefits of eroticism extend beyond the bedroom. Engaging in activities that encourage sensual exploration can boost confidence, enhance body image, and invigorate physiological health. The hormonal balance that is achieved through pleasurable erotic engagement improves overall vitality, supporting the cardiovascular system and enhancing immune response. As a result, one's physical health is not just maintained but flourished.

It is crucial, however, to approach erotic energy with intention and mindfulness. Practising techniques such as deep breathing, meditation, and conscious touch can enhance the way eroticism manifests in our lives, turning ordinary moments into extraordinary experiences. When approached mindfully, these practices cultivate a deeper awareness of the body's responses and its needs, providing insight into our unique erotic landscape.

Ultimately, understanding and harnessing the healing power of eroticism requires a delicate balance. It involves recognising the fluidity of our desires and the boundaries within which we feel comfortable exploring them. By respecting these limits, erotic growth becomes not just about immediate gratification but about a sustainable journey towards overall wellness.

Embracing the healing potential of eroticism opens doors to a more fulfilling existence. It challenges us to see pleasure as a fundamental component of health, encouraging us to integrate erotic energy into our daily lives in meaningful ways. This journey demands courage and self-compassion, as we navigate the intricate dance of desire and fulfilment, yet the rewards are a richer, more vivacious life. Emotional strength, mental clarity, and physical vitality can become the new norm, stemming from a source both ancient and timeless: the profound and empowering power of eroticism.

Chapter 10:
Communication and Desire

In the intricate dance of relationships, communication and desire are inseparable partners, each amplifying and reciprocating the other's rhythms. This chapter delves into the art of communicating openly and effectively, serving as a catalyst for deeper intimacy and enhanced connection. By embracing vulnerability, we unlock a realm where desires can be shared without fear or judgement, fostering an environment ripe for authentic expression and mutual understanding. It's about breaking down barriers and navigating the complex language of emotions, allowing partners to align their intentions and fantasies with kindness and empathy. When words become both shield and bridge, couples can explore the landscape of their desire, discovering the power of dialogue to transform mere interactions into profound engagements of body and spirit. Communication, then, becomes not just a tool but the very heartbeat of desire, guiding us toward a life that's not only fulfilling but vibrantly alive with possibility.

Effective Communication Skills for Intimacy

There's an undeniable power in words, especially when it comes to fostering intimacy. The way we communicate can deeply influence the level of connection and mutual understanding we share with our partners. Effective communication skills become the foundation upon which intimacy is built. With careful and intentional communication, desires are not only expressed but are also heard, respected, and embraced.

The art of communication in intimate relationships often begins with active listening. This isn't just about hearing the words being said; it's about understanding the emotion and intentions behind them. When we truly listen, with empathy and without interruption, we create a safe space for honesty and vulnerability. This kind of listening validates our partner's feelings and experiences, making them feel valued and understood. It involves putting aside our own judgement and entering the conversation with curiosity and open-mindedness.

Equally important in fostering intimacy is the skill of expressing oneself clearly and constructively. Sometimes desires and needs can feel too intimate or risky to voice. Yet, sharing these thoughts with honesty and clarity enriches the relationship. It's about finding the right words and the right tone. Using "I" statements can be incredibly powerful here, as they allow us to express our feelings without casting blame or creating defensiveness. For instance, saying "I feel cherished when you hold my hand" conveys a personal feeling and a specific action, enhancing understanding and emotional closeness.

Non-verbal communication can't be overlooked either. Our body language, facial expressions, and even the pauses between words speak volumes. A gentle touch, eye contact, or a reassuring smile can reinforce what words alone might struggle to convey. Paying attention to these cues, both in ourselves and our partners, amplifies the message we wish to communicate. It underscores sincerity and supports verbal expressions of desire and affection.

Negotiating boundaries is another crucial aspect of communication in intimate relationships. Boundaries aren't walls; they are guidelines that help nurture and protect the relationship. Discussing what each person needs to feel safe and respected can be an intimate experience in itself, fostering deeper trust and understanding.

This isn't a one-time conversation; it should evolve as the relationship grows and as each partner's needs change over time.

Open dialogues about sexual preferences and fantasies can further enrich intimacy. These discussions can initially feel awkward or daunting, especially in relationships where such topics haven't been openly explored. However, approaching these conversations with curiosity and without judgement can lead to profound emotional and sexual intimacy. Sharing fantasies isn't just about what happens in the bedroom; it's about revealing parts of oneself, desires, and vulnerabilities. This exploration should be a joint discovery, fuelled by mutual consent and interest.

Establishing a rhythm of regular check-ins can also maintain and deepen communication. These are not merely opportunities to solve problems but are chances to celebrate the positives in the relationship. They reinforce appreciation and gratitude, focusing on what works well and what each partner values. This positivity sets a loving tone and encourages more open, joyful communication.

At times, external help might be beneficial to bridge communication gaps. Seeking the guidance of a therapist or counsellor can provide valuable insights and techniques, especially when communication feels stuck or fraught with tension. A neutral third party can help identify patterns and suggest practical ways to break them, offering a pathway to reconnecting and communicating more effectively.

In all these aspects, it's crucial to cultivate patience and practice. Building effective communication skills for intimacy doesn't happen overnight. It requires consistent effort, a willingness to learn, and a desire to grow together. It's about striving for understanding over agreement, compassion over criticism, and love over judgement.

By mastering these skills, we not only enhance our intimate relationships but also nurture our own emotional well-being. Effective communication fosters an environment of safety, trust, and mutual respect, which are essential for desire and intimacy to flourish. Embracing this journey equips us with the skills to foster not just a loving relationship but a thriving, dynamic connection filled with passion and understanding.

Understanding and Sharing Desires

Engaging in open communication about desires is a gateway to deeper intimacy and connection. It's akin to peeling back layers of vulnerability, allowing partners to explore and understand each other on a profound level. Speaking openly about what you want and need can feel daunting; societal norms have often shrouded sexual discourse in shame or discomfort. Yet, it is essential for nurturing a fulfilling and balanced life. The courage to express oneself can transform relationships, forging an authentic path to shared joy.

When it comes to sharing your desires, clarity is key. It starts with understanding your own feelings and aspirations. This introspective knowledge lays a foundation for articulating what you want to your partner. Often, desires are clouded by misconceptions or unexpressed emotions. Taking time to reflect can disperse this fog, revealing the core of your true yearnings. It's not just about what happens in the bedroom but encompasses the emotional and physical aspects of the entire relationship.

Consider the dynamics of a relationship where desires are shared openly. Picture how a partner responds not with judgement but with curiosity and empathy. Such conversations can enhance trust and consolidate a team's sense of partnership. They ensure that both individuals feel heard and valued. Understanding requirements doesn't necessarily mean fulfilling all of them, but it involves recognising them as valid and exploring how best to accommodate them within the relationship.

Fostering a communicative environment begins with setting the right tone. Creating a safe space for dialogue is imperative. This means eliminating distractions, actively listening, and responding with understanding rather than defensiveness. Practising this level of communication can feel awkward at first but becomes a natural part of your interaction as partners. Over time, it cultivates a shared language of love and desire that is unique and deeply personal.

Let's not overlook the power of non-verbal communication in expressing desires. Sometimes words might fail to capture the essence of what you're trying to convey. A lingering look, a gentle touch, or a meaningful gesture can speak volumes. Learning to interpret non-verbal cues is equally important, as it helps in reading your partner's needs and desires more accurately. This intuition is sharpened through continuous interaction and attention to detail.

However, sharing desires requires more than just words and actions; it demands an understanding of consensual communication. Both partners must be willing participants in this dialogue. Consent is continual and dynamic, requiring an ongoing conversation where both individuals feel free to express changes in their feelings or boundaries. This mutual respect fosters a healthy environment where desires can be safely explored and negotiated.

The roles that cultural and social influences play in shaping our views on desire cannot be ignored. We often carry within us the narratives of our upbringing, which impacts how we communicate our needs. Acknowledging and discussing these influences can be emancipating. By doing so, partners help each other break free from restrictive norms and embrace a more expansive understanding of their desires.

Meanwhile, the timing of discussions about desires should be considered carefully. Choosing the right moment is crucial. It's best to avoid these conversations during stressful periods or when either partner is preoccupied. Opt for serene settings where both are relaxed and inclined to engage positively. This ensures the conversation is constructive, creating an opportune setting for a deeper connection rather than a potential source of conflict.

Sharing desires is not a one-time affair; it evolves over time. As individuals and circumstances change, desires will also transform. Revisit these conversations regularly—you might discover new aspects of yourself or your partner that were previously unknown. Regular communication reinforces your dedication to the relationship and your commitment to each other's happiness.

The art of sharing desires is not just about sexual needs. It encompasses aspirations, dreams, and the life you wish to build together. Understanding this broader spectrum enhances both physical intimacy and emotional solidarity. When executed thoughtfully, sharing desires reinforces an enduring partnership that thrives not just on compatibility but on a continuously negotiated and shared vision.

In conclusion, embracing the realms of understanding and sharing desires is an invitation to enrich your life and relationships. It demands courage yet offers a reward that's substantial: an enduring, intimate connection that celebrates each individual's needs. As we continue this journey through the labyrinth of sexuality and well-being, remember that every conversation initiated in love and trust is a step towards a more fulfilling existence.

Chapter 11:
Hormones and Sexual Function

In the intricate dance of sexuality, hormones play the role of the silent conductor, orchestrating the rhythms of desire and arousal. These chemical messengers, coursing through our bodies, are pivotal in not only igniting passion but also in maintaining a sense of balance within our sexual function. From the fiery surges of testosterone to the complex interplay of estrogen and oxytocin, each hormone contributes uniquely to the tapestry of sexual experience. Understanding their roles can empower individuals to foster harmony within their bodies. By acknowledging the natural fluctuations that occur throughout different life stages, we can embrace methods to balance these hormones naturally. Whether it's through mindful nutrition, physical activity, or stress management, aligning these forces holistically supports a fulfilling and vibrant sexual life. Through this awareness, we can begin to see how integral our hormonal health is to our overall sense of well-being, inviting us to reassess and rejuvenate our intimate connections in the process.

The Role of Hormones in Desire

In the complex dance of human sexuality, hormones are the oft-hidden musicians whose notes orchestrate desire. While we might often focus on the tangible aspects of sexual attraction and intimacy, the invisible hand of hormones plays a crucial role, intricately weaving together our sexual and overall well-being. They do not act alone or in isolation;

instead, they are part of a delicate system that balances and responds to our environment and inner physical state.

Let's start with testosterone, a name that frequently surfaces in discussions about sexual desire. Though often associated with masculinity, testosterone is a vital component in sexual health for all genders. It's the driving force behind libido for many, influencing motivation, mood, and energy levels. However, it's not just about sheer quantity. The body's sensitivity to this hormone is equally significant. Variations in testosterone levels can affect how one perceives attraction and engagement in intimate encounters.

Oestrogen, predominantly found in higher levels in women, is another powerhouse hormone that contributes to sexual desire. It enhances vaginal lubrication and impacts overall sexual function, making it integral to a pleasurable sexual experience. Fluctuations in oestrogen levels, particularly noticeable during menstruation, pregnancy, or menopause, can significantly alter sexual interest and desire. Its intricate dance with testosterone and progesterone illustrates the delicate balance necessary for sexual desire to flourish.

Speaking of progesterone, this hormone often acts like the unsung hero in the hormonal ensemble. While its role in preparing and maintaining the body for pregnancy is well documented, it also plays a subtle part in regulating mood and sexual desire. During the luteal phase of the menstrual cycle, elevated progesterone levels can lead to decreased libido, a testament to the hormone's profound influence on our sexual landscape.

Dopamine and oxytocin, often referred to as the "feel-good" hormones, are central to our discussion too, closely tied to sexual pleasure and bonding. Dopamine is involved in the reward and pleasure systems of the brain, crucial in the arousal process and the anticipation of sexual activity. Oxytocin, meanwhile, is known as the "cuddle hormone", released during physical intimacy, fostering connection and attachment. Together, they promote a healthy and fulfilling sexual relationship, transcending the physical boundaries and nurturing emotional ties.

Cortisol, commonly known as the stress hormone, can complicate this picture. Chronic stress raises cortisol levels, which can suppress sexual desire and create a cycle of stress and sexual dissatisfaction. It's a prime example of how psychological and physiological states are inextricably linked, underscoring the importance of managing stress in cultivating a thriving sexual life.

Maintaining hormonal balance is key. Our contemporary lifestyle—with its endless demands and stresses—can easily tip this balance, leading to issues with libido. Many find that lifestyle modifications, such as regular exercise, a balanced diet, sufficient sleep, and stress management techniques, work wonders in restoring this equilibrium. When the body is treated well, the hormones find their natural rhythm, and this harmony is often reflected in one's sexual desire and function.

The interplay between hormones and desire is further influenced by life stages and personal circumstances. Puberty marks the onset of hormonal awakening, setting the stage for burgeoning sexuality. Pregnancy and postpartum periods bring profound hormonal changes, affecting sexual interest in unique ways for each individual. Menopause heralds another significant shift, often requiring a re-evaluation of sexual health strategies to adjust to changing hormonal landscapes.

Exploring the role of hormones in sexual desire leads to a greater appreciation of our intricate biology. It's enlightening to consider how these chemical messengers affect not just our bodies but our connections with others. Acknowledging and understanding this can empower individuals to embrace their sexual health as a central aspect of a well-rounded, healthy life.

Through the lens of hormones, we can see how nurturing sexual health is about more than addressing problems when they arise; it's about fostering a proactive and informed approach to our overall well-being. Recognising the importance of these hormonal players offers a pathway to understanding not only what drives desire but also what hinders it. This knowledge demystifies the often unpredictable nature of libido, offering a foundation upon which individuals can build a more conscious and fulfilling sexual existence.

As science continues to unravel more about hormones and their effects, we find ourselves at the cusp of a new understanding of sexual health. This ongoing exploration calls on us to remain curious, considerate, and compassionate about our body's natural rhythms and the powerful voice of hormones in the symphony of desire.

Balancing Hormones Naturally

The intricate dance of hormones within our bodies is nothing short of a symphony that orchestrates our sexual function and overall well-being. It's fascinating how these chemical messengers operate quietly yet powerfully influencing everything from mood to metabolism and libido. When it comes to sexual health, the role of hormones is critical. But here's the silver lining: there are ways to support and balance these hormones naturally, bringing harmony to this complex system.

Understanding the connection between hormones and sexual function involves recognising the major players, such as oestrogen, testosterone, and progesterone—all of which have prominent roles in maintaining sexual health. Each of these hormones has its own unique function, but collectively they work to regulate desire, sexual performance, and fertility. When the balance tilts, it can lead to issues such as reduced libido, erectile dysfunction, or irregular menstrual cycles. Fortunately, adopting natural strategies can help in recalibrating these hormones.

One of the most effective ways to naturally balance hormones is through diet. Eating a balanced diet rich in whole foods provides the nutrients that the body needs to produce and regulate hormones adequately. Foods high in omega-3 fatty acids, such as flaxseeds, walnuts, and oily fish, support hormone production and reduce inflammation. Cruciferous vegetables like broccoli and kale have compounds that assist the liver in detoxifying excess hormones. Including these in your meals regularly can lay a strong foundation for hormonal health.

In addition to diet, exercise plays a significant role in balancing hormones. Regular physical activity improves insulin sensitivity, lowers stress hormones like cortisol, and helps maintain a healthy weight—all factors that contribute to harmonious hormone levels. Whether it's through brisk walking, yoga, or lifting weights, staying active is a natural and effective way to manage your hormonal health. Plus, exercise releases endorphins, which can buoy mood and indirectly boost sexual desire.

Stress management is another pillar of maintaining hormonal balance. Chronic stress can wreak havoc on hormonal harmony by spiking cortisol levels, which in turn can suppress thyroid function and reduce the production of sex hormones. Incorporating relaxation techniques such as meditation, deep-breathing exercises, or spending time in nature can mitigate stress and support a more balanced hormonal landscape.

Sleep is often an overlooked element in the hormonal equation. The body's hormonal network requires consistent and adequate rest to function optimally. During the sleep cycle, particularly in deep REM, the body works to repair cells and regulate hormone production. Aiming for 7-9 hours of quality sleep each night can significantly impact hormone levels, leading to improved sexual function and overall well-being.

Herbal remedies have also been embraced as natural allies in the quest for hormonal balance. For example, maca root is known for its ability to bolster energy and sexual desire in both men and women. Similarly, herbs such as ashwagandha and ginseng have adaptogenic properties, meaning they help the body adapt to stress and stabilise hormone levels. Incorporating these herbs into your routine, whether through teas or supplements, can provide gentle support for hormone health.

Moreover, ensuring that your environment is conducive to hormonal health is crucial. This means minimising exposure to endocrine disruptors—chemicals found in plastics, pesticides, and even personal care products—that can interfere with hormone function. Opting for organic produce, using glass instead of plastic, and choosing natural beauty products can reduce the body's burden of these harmful chemicals.

Connecting with others and fostering emotional intimacy are often underestimated in their power to harmonise hormones. Positive interpersonal relationships can increase the release of oxytocin, the 'love hormone,' which not only enhances feelings of pleasure and connection but also counteracts the stress response, promoting overall hormonal balance.

Finally, regular health check-ups cannot be overstated. Periodic evaluations by a healthcare professional can help monitor hormone levels and identify any imbalances early on. This proactive approach allows for timely interventions, whether through lifestyle changes or other therapies, to safeguard against potential issues.

In conclusion, the journey to balance hormones naturally is a holistic one. It invites us to weave together elements of nutrition, movement, rest, stress reduction, and connection. By aligning these aspects of life, we create a robust framework for enhancing sexual function and nurturing our overall well-being. Remember that small, consistent changes can lead to significant transformations, leaving you empowered to embrace a more harmonious state of health.

Chapter 12:
Exploring Sexual Identity

In this chapter, we embark on a journey to understand the multifaceted nature of sexual identity, an essential part of our overall well-being. Sexual identity is not a static label but a vibrant spectrum, offering a colourful tapestry of possibilities for self-expression and understanding. Recognising and embracing one's unique sexual self can lead to profound personal growth, enhancing relationships, and fostering a deeper sense of belonging. Exploring this dimension of identity invites self-reflection and courage, as it often challenges societal norms and personal boundaries. As we navigate through the spectrum of sexual identities, we uncover the transformative power of authenticity and acceptance, celebrating diversity in all its forms. This chapter encourages embracing this exploration with an open heart, empowering each individual to contribute to a more inclusive and compassionate world.

The Spectrum of Sexual Identities

Sexual identity is an expansive and diverse realm, embodying the intricate facets that form our attractions, orientations, and self-perceptions. It's a tapestry, woven from the threads of personal experience and cultural background, yet distinctively individual for each person. Understanding this spectrum is pivotal for embracing one's sexual self, contributing not only to personal well-being but also forging deeper connections with others.

The notion of sexuality goes beyond the binary framework of heterosexuality and homosexuality. It encompasses a rich spectrum of identities including bisexuality, pansexuality, asexuality, and many more. Each of these identities holds its own unique experiences and perspectives. Appreciating the breadth of sexual identities means acknowledging the validity and importance of everyone's personal journey and understanding the freedom to explore these paths without the constraints of societal norms.

Among these identities, bisexuality often illustrates the fluidity of attraction. It's painted by a palette of interests that don't necessarily fit into the singular categorisation of 'gay' or 'straight'. The versatility of bisexuality can be liberating, yet societal myths may create challenges for those identifying as bisexual, suggesting they exist in a state of 'indecision'. Recognising the intrinsic legitimacy of bisexuality without judgement is a step towards a more inclusive understanding of sexual identities.

Pansexuality broadens this scope further, recognising attraction irrespective of gender. Unlike bisexuality, which traditionally acknowledges two or more genders, pansexuality embraces an attraction to people across the entire gender continuum. This conceptualisation emphasises that love and attraction transcend gender binaries, reinforcing the idea that emotional and sexual connections are multi-faceted and boundless.

Asexuality represents another vital part of the spectrum, where individuals may not experience sexual attraction at all. This identity often challenges societal views that equate sexual desire with love or relationship fulfilment. Asexual individuals navigate their identities in a world that often prioritises and emphasises sexual attraction as a marker of normalcy. Understanding asexuality involves reconceptualising attraction and relationship dynamics, underlining the diversity in human connections and affection.

Many people ponder where they 'fit' on this spectrum. The idea of fitting in, however, is an antiquated notion. Sexual identity isn't stagnant; it's a dynamic, evolving aspect of ourselves that can shift over time. It's not uncommon for someone to identify differently at various stages of their life depending on personal experiences and self-discovery. This fluidity should be celebrated as part of individual authenticity and growth.

For some, exploring sexual identity is a deeply personal journey that can involve significant introspection and, sometimes, external challenges. Fear of rejection or misunderstanding by peers, family, or society at large can cause an internal conflict that impacts mental and emotional well-being. Yet, understanding one's sexual identity can be empowering, enabling individuals to align with their true self and foster genuine connections with others.

Communication plays a crucial role in embracing and expressing one's sexual identity. Open, honest conversations about feelings and attractions can facilitate greater acceptance and understanding from those around us. Encouraging dialogue that honours and respects each person's unique experiences helps to dismantle stereotypes and prejudices, making space for inclusivity.

When we start to explore these identities, we enter into a narrative of possibilities. Everyone's story contributes to the wider discourse on sexuality and well-being. Within this spectrum, language and terminologies are constantly evolving to give voice to shared and individual experiences. This linguistic evolution not only reflects changes in the way identities are viewed but also validates diverse existences and their place within society.

In supporting individuals as they explore and affirm their identities, allied communities serve as vital spaces. They provide a supportive environment that's free from judgment, fostering interaction and education that enriches the broader social fabric. This sense of community can offer a haven where people feel seen and understood, which is central to their happiness and confidence.

Systems and policies, too, need to adapt to acknowledge and protect the rights of those across the sexual identity spectrum. It's about ensuring equality and freedom from discrimination in all areas of life—from employment to healthcare, and education to personal relationships. These systems must make room for flexibility, recognising the multitude of ways in which identities can manifest.

It's also critical to address internalised stereotypes and prejudices that individuals may carry, knowingly or unknowingly. By actively engaging with and challenging such biases, we nurture an environment where acceptance is the norm, not the exception. This acts as a catalyst for individual enlightenment and broader societal change.

The intersectionality of sexual identities with other aspects of identity, including race, culture, and religion, adds layers of complexity. These intersections shape how people experience their sexual identities and the unique challenges they face. By acknowledging these intersections, there's room to create more nuanced and supportive frameworks that consider the whole person.

A truly holistic understanding embraces the idea that every person's journey is valid. Empowerment comes not just from recognising one's own identity but from valuing the identities and experiences of others. By highlighting the diversity within the spectrum of sexual identities, we cultivate a society where everyone can thrive, leading to a more fulfilling, joyous existence.

In the grand tapestry of human experience, sexual identities shape how we relate to each other and ourselves. Recognising the spectrum is not about compartmentalising individuals into defined categories, but about celebrating the vibrant array of human expression. By doing so, we pave the way for greater understanding, love, and respect, nurturing the well-being of individuals and society as a whole.

Embracing One's Sexual Self

For many, embracing one's sexual self is akin to embarking on a profound journey, full of discovery, acceptance, and growth. It's about peeling back the layers society has wrapped around sexuality and finding the authentic self beneath. This journey can be both exhilarating and challenging, requiring a willingness to confront existing perceptions and embrace new understandings of one's sexual identity.

Sexual identity is often shaped by a web of influences, from familial and cultural expectations to personal experiences and societal norms. Many people start this exploration with the realization that their sexual identity might not fit neatly into preconceived categories. This process, though initially daunting, offers an opportunity to delve deeper into what one truly desires and how they define themselves.

To embrace one's sexual self fully, first, there's a need to acknowledge the past without judgment. Consider this: all experiences, whether affirming or challenging, have contributed to the present understanding. It's about looking back without regret, recognising the lessons learned from previous encounters and decisions, and using them as stepping stones to move forward. Acceptance allows individuals to see the beauty in their journey, finding value even in the missteps.

Embracing one's sexual self often initiates a dialogue between mind and body. To foster this conversation, one can explore the sensations and emotions tied to sexual experiences. It's crucial to listen to the body's responses—what feels invigorating, comforting, or exciting—and reflect on these sensations. Mindfulness plays a key role here, helping individuals to stay present, fostering a deeper awareness of genuine desires, and cultivating a sense of harmony between mind and body.

Furthermore, understanding the spectrum of sexual identities can liberate individuals from restrictive labels. It's a broad spectrum that recognises fluidity and change. Embracing fluidity means accepting that identity may evolve over time; what feels right today may shift tomorrow, and that's alright. This openness to change is crucial, allowing for authentic self-expression without the fear of judgment or the need to conform to outdated paradigms.

Confidence naturally follows acceptance. When individuals feel at ease with their sexual identity, it radiates outward, influencing interactions and relationships positively. A confident individual is more likely to engage openly with partners, expressing desires and boundaries clearly, and cultivating healthier, more satisfying relationships. This newfound self-assurance can transform not just sexual relationships but every aspect of life, fostering a fuller, richer experience of the world.

The path to embracing one's sexual self isn't solitary. Connections with others who share similar experiences or understandings can be incredibly affirming. Communities that celebrate diversity in sexual identities offer support and can provide a space to share stories and experiences. This network of support can be a powerful motivator, encouraging individuals to continue on their journeys with courage and resilience.

In embracing one's sexual self, there is immense power in storytelling—not just to others, but to oneself. Reflecting on personal narratives helps in recognising patterns, uncovering truths, and dismantling myths that have long held power. It's an exercise in vulnerability that cultivates strength, acknowledging where one has been while consciously choosing the path forward.

Naturally, embracing one's sexual self—or even starting this exploration—comes with challenges. Socio-cultural norms and prejudices can be formidable, creating internal conflicts and external pressures. Overcoming these obstacles requires perseverance and often, the courage to challenge the status quo. Yet, by leaning on a robust support network and utilising educational resources, individuals can navigate these hurdles with greater ease.

Create a personal space, both physically and emotionally, for exploration. Whether through journaling, meditation, or conversation with trusted allies, dedicate time to understanding and nurturing one's sexual self. This personal sanctuary serves as a reminder of the commitment to self-acceptance and growth, providing refuge and strength during moments of doubt.

Nurturing one's sexual self can also involve creative explorations. Engage in activities that resonate with personal desires and interests, whether through art, dance, or any other form of expression. Creativity can be a conduit for revealing hidden aspects of one's identity and fostering an environment where the sexual self is free to flourish without restriction.

Through this journey, never underestimate the power of seeking professional guidance. Therapists and counsellors who specialise in sexual identity can offer invaluable insights and strategies, helping individuals navigate the complex emotions and experiences that arise. They provide a safe space for individuals to explore their sexual identities without judgment, aiding in the process of integration and acceptance.

The rewards of embracing one's sexual self are vast, leading to a more authentic and fulfilling existence. By integrating this aspect of identity into everyday life, individuals experience an overall sense of wellbeing. The journey, while personal, is also universal—one that highlights the interconnectedness of sexual health and holistic well-being.

As this exploration unfolds, remember that identity is not a destination but a continuous journey. Embracing one's sexual self is about honouring the journey, understanding that it's unique for each individual. The ultimate goal is to integrate sexual identity as a vital aspect of one's overall well-being, leading to enriched relationships and a balanced life. Embrace the exploration and cherish the process, for it is through this journey that true self-acceptance and fulfilment are found.

Chapter 13:
Ageing and Sexuality

Ageing gracefully doesn't mean the fading of sexual vitality, but rather an evolution of intimacy and desire. As people journey through various life stages, the shifting landscape of sexuality demands embracing new experiences and perspectives. With age, sexual expression takes on a more nuanced form, enriched by wisdom and deepened connections. Navigating the challenges posed by ageing—such as hormonal changes and societal perceptions—can empower individuals to maintain a fulfilling and dynamic sexual life. It's about recognising that the essence of sexuality transforms but never loses its inherent power. By staying attuned to both the body's signals and emotional needs, people can overcome barriers and foster a passionate, authentic sexual identity at every age. In essence, the golden years can shine with potent sensuality when approached with openness and adaptability, celebrating the longevity of sexual wellness as a journey rather than a retreat.

Maintaining Desire Across the Lifespan

As we traverse through life, our relationship with desire evolves alongside the many milestones we encounter. A vibrant and fulfilling sexual life is intricately connected to our overall well-being, contributing to both our physical health and emotional satisfaction. Yet, the journey of maintaining desire across the lifespan can be complex, requiring a nuanced understanding of the various factors that influence our sexual vitality as we age.

The natural process of ageing brings with it changes that can impact sexual desire, but these changes don't have to mean a decline in sexual satisfaction. Instead, they offer an opportunity to explore new dimensions of intimacy and connection. Keeping desire alive means remaining open to the evolution of sexuality and adapting to the shifts that come with different life stages. This adaptability nurtures not only individual health but also the health of relationships, fostering deeper connections that are characterised by understanding and empathy.

Understanding the Fluid Nature of Sexual Desire Desire isn't a static entity; it ebbs and flows, shaped by both internal factors like hormones and external influences such as stress and lifestyle changes. Recognising the fluid nature of sexual desire empowers individuals to embrace change rather than fear it. With openness comes a deeper appreciation for the body's capacity to experience pleasure and intimacy, leading to a more nuanced understanding of one's sexual self.

With age, the body undergoes physiological changes that can alter experiences of desire and arousal. Hormonal shifts, particularly during menopause and andropause, can lead to decreased libido. However, these changes should not signal the end of a fulfilling sexual life. Instead, they can serve as a catalyst for exploring new avenues of intimacy and pleasure. By focusing on emotional intimacy and mutual exploration, many find their connections with their partners deepen, revealing new layers of attraction and desire.

The Role of Communication in Sustaining Desire Open and honest communication becomes increasingly crucial in maintaining desire across the lifespan. Conversations about needs, preferences, and fears create a respectful space to address concerns that arise with age. This open dialogue can enhance intimacy and understanding, bridging the gaps that years of routine and familiarity might create.

Sharing experiences and being willing to adapt are key to sustaining a vibrant sexual connection. It's essential to consider both partners' perspectives and to approach changes with patience and creativity. This collaborative stance not only keeps the spark alive but also reinforces the emotional bonds that support enduring relationships.

Embracing New Modes of Exploration Ageing can be an invitation to reimagine the ways in which we experience desire and sexual fulfilment. Many find that this stage in life allows for a greater focus on sensuality and emotional intimacy, moving beyond the physical to a more holistic experience. Discovering pleasure in the subtle, everyday connections can lead to a richer, more fulfilling sexual life.

Incorporating new practices, such as mindfulness or tantric techniques, can invigorate one's sexual experience. These practices help individuals connect with their bodies in new ways, enhancing sensitivity and awareness. The journey of discovery continues, inviting a reconsideration of what it means to be sexually vibrant at different ages.

Physical Health and Its Impact on Desire Maintaining physical health is a cornerstone of sustaining sexual desire. Regular exercise, a balanced diet, and adequate sleep contribute significantly to sexual vitality. These elements become increasingly important as we age, supporting both desire and performance.

Regular physical activity not only improves physical health but also boosts mood and energy levels, helping to counteract the effects of ageing on sexual desire. Exercises that promote flexibility and strength, such as yoga, can also enhance body awareness and contribute to a positive sexual outlook. Additionally, maintaining a healthy diet rich in essential nutrients like antioxidants and amino acids supports hormone balance and energy levels.

Psychological and Emotional Well-being Emotional health is intertwined with sexual desire, influencing our ability to experience and express intimacy. As people age, experiences such as loss, stress, and shifts in identity can impact emotional well-being. Addressing these psychological components is essential in maintaining a healthy sexual life.

Cultivating a positive mental attitude, managing stress, and dealing with emotional blockages can significantly enhance one's capacity for intimacy and desire. Practising mindfulness and self-care can mitigate negative impacts, offering a path towards resilience and sustenance in one's sexual journey.

Celebrating the Wisdom of Age The experience and wisdom that come with age can bring a new level of depth and richness to sexual relationships. There's a beauty in the familiarity that long-term partners share, where deeper emotional connections create a unique bond. The ability to communicate desires and share intimate moments without fear or inhibition celebrates the journey of life and love.

Each stage of life presents its own challenges and opportunities. Embracing change and growth in sexuality allows for a continuous journey of desire and enjoyment. It's about celebrating the present moment, respecting the past, and looking forward to new experiences with hope and enthusiasm. While ageing may alter certain aspects of sexual desire, it certainly doesn't have to diminish the joy and vitality of a loving and satisfying sexual connection.

Overcoming Age-related Challenges

Ageing is an inevitable journey, but it does not necessarily mean the demise of sexual desire or satisfaction. Indeed, embracing sexuality as an integral part of our lives must include recognising and overcoming the challenges that ageing presents. Changes in sexual health with age are natural, but understanding and navigating them are crucial for maintaining intimacy and connection at any stage of life.

The body undergoes a myriad of physiological changes as it ages, many of which can affect sexual health. The decrease in hormone levels, such as oestrogen and testosterone, often leads to a sheer dip in libido. Women may encounter vaginal dryness or atrophy due to menopause, while men might experience erectile dysfunction more frequently. However, these changes don't have to be barriers to a fulfilling sexual life. Treatments and therapies are available to help tackle these issues, ranging from hormone replacement treatments to the use of lubricants or medications.

Purely physical factors aren't the only ones in play; mental and emotional health is inextricably linked to sexual well-being. As people grow older, they may face emotional issues such as depression, anxiety, or worries about ageing itself, impacting their desire and performance. Addressing these feelings openly, perhaps through counselling or therapy, is a positive step towards reconciling one's sexual identity with the ageing process. A healthy mindset contributes to a healthy sex life, underscoring the importance of mental wellness in tackling age-related sexual challenges.

Aging is also a time when couples can encounter changes in their relationships, such as empty nesting or retirement, which alter the dynamic of daily living. These transitions can offer an opportunity to rediscover each other sexually. Engaging openly in communication about desires and boundaries can rekindle intimacy. Couples are encouraged to approach these years as a time for exploration and adaptation rather than resistance to change.

Incorporating physical activities and maintaining a balanced diet go hand in hand with sexual health at any age. Exercise improves circulation, which is crucial for sexual arousal and performance. It also enhances mood and body image, both of which are essential for a vibrant sexual life. Moreover, a diet rich in nutrients supports hormone production and energy levels, contributing to overall vitality and sexual function. Tailoring fitness and nutrition to fit one's changing body needs can keep the spark alive.

Moreover, the experience that comes with age can be an advantage. Older individuals often have a clearer understanding of their own bodies and what brings them pleasure. This knowledge allows for more confident expression in intimate situations. The maturity that aging provides can serve as a powerful tool in achieving gratifying sexual encounters.

Societal perceptions of sexual activity among older adults often come with stigma and misunderstanding. Overcoming these misconceptions involves challenging stereotypes and acknowledging that sexuality doesn't fade with age—it evolves. Encouraging open dialogue and education about ageing and sexuality within communities can foster a more inclusive environment, empowering older adults to embrace their sexual identities without shame or suspicion.

Indeed, some individuals find that their sex lives improve as they grow older, experiencing a new type of freedom. With potentially fewer responsibilities, such as child-rearing or career pressures, many find they have more time and energy to devote to their sexual relationships. The golden years can be a time of sexual enlightenment when approached with a sense of curiosity and adaptability.

Embracing these shifts can be akin to embarking on a new adventure. It's vital to adopt an attitude that views these changes as part of the normal ageing process rather than roadblocks to pleasure. Developing patience, both with oneself and with one's partner, allows for the necessary adjustments that can lead to continued fulfillment and satisfaction.

Valuing sexual health is more important than ever as we age. It not only contributes to overall happiness and well-being but also has positive effects on physical health, such as improved heart health and a strengthened immune system. By prioritising sexual health throughout life's changes, older adults can enjoy these benefits, enriching their quality of life and longevity.

The journey doesn't end as we age; it pivots towards new possibilities and deeper connections. Remaining tuned into one's physical and emotional needs, while embracing a proactive approach, can overcome the age-related challenges that arise in sexual health. It's about understanding, adjusting, and ultimately celebrating this intrinsic aspect of human experience, allowing it to flourish at every stage of life.

Chapter 14:
Overcoming Sexual Dysfunction

In the intricate dance of intimacy, sexual dysfunction can feel like a stumbling block, yet acknowledging its presence is the first step towards healing and rediscovery. This chapter peels back the layers of what often feels isolating, revealing a pathway towards understanding and resolution. By approaching this issue with both curiosity and compassion, one learns that overcoming sexual dysfunction isn't solely about seeking fixes—it's about reconnecting with one's own needs and desires in a more profound way. Mental resilience plays a pivotal role, as unravelling entrenched beliefs and anxieties can liberate one's innate capacity for pleasure. Techniques such as therapy and mindfulness can foster a sense of control and rejuvenation, turning challenges into opportunities for growth. By leaning into vulnerability and embracing open dialogues, individuals can transform obstacles into bridges, leading to enriched relationships and an enhanced sense of self. This journey through dysfunction can teach us that sexual well-being is not just a goal but an integral part of a nurturing and vibrant life.

Common Sexual Disorders and Their Solutions

Sexual dysfunction can cast a long shadow over one's personal life, affecting both individuals and couples in profound ways. These common sexual disorders are not just physical conditions; they intertwine with emotional and mental well-being, often creating a complex web that's challenging to unravel. However, armed with the right knowledge and a proactive mindset, it's possible to navigate these obstacles and come out the other side with a deeper understanding of oneself and one's relational dynamics.

One of the most prevalent sexual disorders is erectile dysfunction (ED), which affects an alarming number of individuals globally. Often linked with an array of underlying medical conditions such as diabetes, cardiovascular disease, and hypertension, ED is also heavily influenced by psychological factors, including stress and anxiety. The solution begins with open communication and medical consultation, focusing on addressing any root causes. In many cases, lifestyle modifications, such as regular exercise and a heart-healthy diet, can significantly improve symptoms. For some, medication or alternative therapies may be prescribed, though psychological support and counselling often play a crucial role in long-term healing.

Similarly, female sexual arousal disorder (FSAD) is another common issue that, unfortunately, is often overlooked. This condition, characterised by a lack of sexual arousal and interest, can stem from hormonal imbalances, previous trauma, or relational issues. Solutions here involve multi-faceted approaches such as hormonal therapy, if appropriate, and therapeutic interventions focusing on improving self-esteem and fostering emotional connections with partners. Incorporating mindfulness techniques and focusing on increasing emotional and physical intimacy can equally be beneficial, promoting a nurturing space for sexual exploration and growth.

Premature ejaculation is another widespread concern, affecting men across all ages. The root causes can vary from psychological factors such as performance anxiety to biological triggers like unusual hormone levels. Addressing premature ejaculation often involves a combination of behavioural techniques, like the "stop-start" method or "squeeze" technique, which can retrain the body's responses. Psychological support may also be incorporated to alleviate anxiety or stressors contributing to the condition. The journey requires patience, but with determination and often the support of a professional, long-lasting solutions can be found.

A condition that receives less attention but is no less impactful is hypoactive sexual desire disorder (HSDD), affecting both men and women. Characterised by a chronic lack of interest in sex, it's often linked with hormonal imbalances, life stresses, or even partner relationship issues. In treating HSDD, understanding the underpinning emotional or psychological factors is vital. Psychological counselling or sex therapy often serves as a beneficial avenue, helping individuals and couples enhance their sexual communication, set realistic expectations, and foster intimacy. Hormonal treatments can also play a supportive role when appropriate, but the crux lies in reviving sexual spontaneity and joy.

Painful intercourse, medically known as dyspareunia, is another barrier to sexual fulfilment, commonly affecting women but also impacting some men. This condition might originate from physical causes such as infections, endometriosis, or menopause-related changes. Solutions involve medical treatments to resolve physical issues and may be complemented by pelvic floor therapy to relax and strengthen muscles. Emotional support can empower individuals to navigate feelings of anxiety or fear that often accompany this condition, gradually restoring confidence and comfort in sexual experiences.

Beyond these dominant issues, other disorders such as delayed ejaculation, orgasmic disorder, and vaginismus present unique challenges. While the origins can be quite varied—from physical conditions and medication side effects to deeply entrenched psychological blocks—comprehensive and personalised approaches are key. For instance, orgasmic disorder might benefit from explorations into one's sexual script and expectations, while vaginismus could require both physical therapy and extensive psychological support. Each path to resolution is as unique as the individual experiencing the condition.

These common sexual disorders have solutions that illuminate a broader truth for anyone affected by them or by any other sexual health issue—a holistic approach is essential. Treating symptoms in isolation seldom leads to lasting change. Instead, recognising and addressing intertwined physical, emotional, and relational dimensions invariably paves a more successful path to recovery. Encouragement and understanding from partners, alongside professional guidance, create a nurturing environment where healing can thrive.

The journey through sexual dysfunction is personal and often complex, laden with emotional and psychological intricacies. However, by breaking the silence surrounding these issues and seeking comprehensive strategies tailored to individual needs, recovery and rejuvenation are entirely within reach. With effort and patience, these challenges can lead to newfound depths of personal and relational satisfaction, cementing the essential role of sexual health in our overall well-being.

Mental Approaches to Healing Dysfunction

When it comes to overcoming sexual dysfunction, the role of the mind cannot be overstated. Mental approaches to healing dysfunction offer a path to rediscovering one's sexual vitality and embracing a fulfilling intimate life. These strategies delve deeply into the psyche, seeking to dismantle barriers and reveal the boundless potential for pleasure and connection that resides within every individual. The journey begins with understanding the profound connection between one's mind and sexual function.

Recognising the root causes of sexual dysfunction often involves introspection. Anxiety, depression, and stress are frequent culprits that hinder sexual health. These emotional states can create a self-perpetuating cycle where fear of sexual inadequacy leads to performance anxiety, which, in turn, exacerbates dysfunction. Breaking this cycle requires adopting a mindset geared towards change and growth, where one learns to embrace vulnerability and acknowledge that these challenges are not immutable.

Mindfulness is an invaluable tool in this mental repertoire. By fostering a sense of presence, individuals can tune into their bodies and emotions, letting go of worries about past performance or future outcomes. Mindfulness meditation, for instance, cultivates an awareness that encourages individuals to savour each moment and sensation, enhancing their capacity for pleasure. The practice involves focusing on the present, recognising and accepting thoughts without judgement, which helps diminish anxiety and enhances sexual experience.

Another pivotal mental approach is cognitive behavioural therapy (CBT). CBT assists individuals in identifying and altering negative thought patterns that contribute to sexual dysfunction. It is a structured, goal-oriented form of psychotherapy, focusing on the interplay between thoughts, emotions, and behaviours. Within this context, therapy encourages new cognitive strategies to reinterpret sexual experiences positively, bypassing obstacles rooted in past trauma or ingrained misconceptions about sexuality.

Self-compassion and acceptance play a crucial role as well. It's essential to counteract self-critical thoughts with kindness and understanding. Embracing one's own imperfections can alleviate the pressure to perform, paving the way for genuine intimacy and connection. Self-compassion practices can include simple affirmations and reflective journaling, both aimed at cultivating a nurturing, non-judgemental relationship with oneself, thus allowing for a more relaxed and pleasurable sexual expression.

Visualisation techniques can also be exceedingly beneficial. Through guided imagery or erotic fantasies, individuals can explore their sexuality in a safe and controlled manner. This practice empowers the mind to transcend its limitations, opening up new avenues for arousal and intimacy. Visualisation isn't about creating expectations but rather about tapping into personal desires and expanding one's comfort zone within the realm of sexual experience.

Reframing sexual dysfunction not as a personal failing but as a signal of underlying issues offers liberation from the stigma and shame often associated with these challenges. This shift in perspective can cultivate a sense of agency, empowering individuals to seek personalised strategies for healing. Sexual dysfunction is not an identity but a condition, and with appropriate mental approaches, it can be addressed effectively.

Developing a personalised goal-oriented plan in collaboration with a mental health professional can provide a roadmap for recovery. This plan might incorporate elements of all the aforementioned approaches, tailored to the unique needs of the individual. A therapist can help to chart progress, adjust strategies, and celebrate achievements, offering support and encouragement throughout the healing journey.

Moreover, fostering open communication with partners is vital. Sharing fears, desires, and aspirations within a relationship can fortify bonds and create a supportive environment for sexual exploration and healing. Vulnerability in communication fosters empathy and understanding, counteracting isolation and emphasising mutual respect and care.

Lastly, educational efforts to demystify sexual health are paramount. By understanding anatomy, physiology, and the complexities of desire, individuals can alleviate fears borne of ignorance or misconceptions. Knowledge equips individuals with the confidence to challenge and reframe dysfunction, empowering them to navigate their sexual health with informed agency and competence.

In conclusion, mental approaches to healing sexual dysfunction offer a nuanced and holistic path to sexual well-being. By embracing mindfulness, cognitive restructuring, self-compassion, and open dialogue, individuals can overcome barriers and cultivate a fulfilling and vibrant sexual life. This journey is a testament to the indomitable resilience of the human spirit, highlighting the transformative power of the mind in reclaiming intimacy and connection.

Chapter 15:
Spiritual Aspects of Sexuality

Spirituality and sexuality are intertwined realms, offering a profound union that can enhance both personal and shared life experiences. By recognising the spiritual dimensions of our sexual selves, we embark on a journey that transcends physical pleasure and penetrates the very essence of our being. This harmony invites a deeper connection, not just with ourselves but also with our partners and the universe. Practices such as tantra and mindfulness guide us toward a more sacred form of intimacy where vulnerability and trust become gateways to spiritual awakening. In nurturing this bond, we unlock new levels of fulfilment, rooted in authenticity and compassion. As we explore these spiritual aspects, we find that sexual expression adds layers of meaning to our existence, revealing a path to holistic well-being and a more enriched life. Here, spirituality doesn't overshadow sexuality; instead, it illuminates its beauty, making every shared moment an act of reverence and love.

The Connection between Sexuality and Spirituality

Deep within the human experience, an intricate dance exists between sexuality and spirituality. These two realms, often perceived as distinct, intertwine in profound ways that can be transformative and healing. In many traditions, sexuality is viewed not merely as a biological drive or a pursuit of pleasure, but as a pathway to spiritual awakening. It's an avenue through which people can experience a deeper connection with themselves, others, and even the universe.

Sexuality, at its core, is an expression of creative energy. It's this creativity that invites us to explore who we are, beyond social constructs and limitations. In spiritual contexts, this energy is often linked to concepts like life force or chi, surrounding our very essence and being. When channeled with intention, sexual energy can open doors to higher states of consciousness, enabling individuals to explore dimensions of their spirituality they might never have accessed otherwise.

The relationship between sexuality and spirituality is echoed throughout history and across various cultures. In ancient Hindu and Buddhist traditions, practices such as Tantra teach the harmonisation of spiritual and sexual energies. Tantric principles suggest that by embracing our sexual nature, we can foster a deeper connection with the divine. This integration of sex and soul can lead to a more holistic sense of well-being, highlighting our interconnectedness with the greater cosmos.

Beyond ancient philosophies, many modern spiritual practitioners advocate for integrating these aspects of identity as a way of achieving balance. The process involves recognising sexual experiences as more than physical acts; they are spiritual exchanges that offer insights into our innermost selves. Through this mindful engagement with sexuality, individuals often discover latent potentials within themselves: the capacity for profound love, compassion, and joy. By perceiving sexual energy as sacred, it becomes possible to transform ordinary experiences into extraordinary moments of spiritual insight and growth.

Some might wonder, how does one begin to explore this intersection? One approach is through heightened awareness and presence. Mindfulness practices can play a crucial role in bridging the gap between sexuality and spirituality. By staying present and fully engaged during sexual experiences, individuals can cultivate a deeper sense of connection, not just to their partner but also to the spiritual dimensions of their being. This mindfulness can transform physical encounters into spiritual rituals, paving the way for enlightenment and ecstasy.

It's worth noting that integrating spirituality and sexuality is not about perfection or idealisation. It's about embracing the messy, beautiful complexity of human experience. Perhaps it's in imperfections that the most authentic spirituality emerges. In learning to accept and love oneself entirely, including one's sexual nature, it becomes possible to reach deeper levels of compassion and understanding for all things.

However, this journey can come with its challenges. Social and cultural influences may present barriers to a harmonious connection between sexuality and spirituality. Many carry stigmas and taboos around sexual expression, which can foster shame or guilt. These emotions are detrimental to spiritual well-being, creating internal divisions rather than unity. Overcoming these barriers requires courage and openness to redefine one's identity beyond societal expectations, focussing instead on inner truth and personal experience.

As individuals journey through life, embracing the connection between sexuality and spirituality can lead to profound transformations. This integration encourages the discovery of a more expansive sense of self, one that transcends the mundane to touch the sacred. In this higher state of consciousness, personal growth flourishes, ultimately leading to greater satisfaction and fulfillment in all areas of life.

For those seeking to embrace this path, practices such as meditation, conscious breathing, and body awareness can facilitate a more profound spiritual experience of sexuality. Engaging in such practices doesn't only enhance physical sensations but also invites a deeper introspection about one's spiritual nature. This process can offer insights and revelations that positively influence how individuals view themselves and their connections to others.

Through understanding the connection between sexuality and spirituality, people can achieve a more balanced, integrated existence. By perceiving sexual energy as a spiritual resource, one can break free from the limitations imposed by purely physical perceptions of intimacy. This shift allows us to see sexuality as a sacred offering, a way to celebrate our existence and our place within the universe's grand tapestry.

In conclusion, the journey to unify sexuality and spirituality is deeply personal, rich with potential for growth and transformation. It challenges individuals to explore the depths of their being while expanding their understanding of what it means to be alive and connected to everything around them. This path is a journey worth taking, as it promises a life of greater harmony, fulfilment, and spiritual awakening.

Practices for Spiritual Sexual Intimacy

In the realm of human experience, sexuality and spirituality are often seen as separate, even conflicting dimensions. Yet, by weaving these two aspects together, we can discover a richer, more profound connection not only with our partners but also with ourselves. Embracing practices that integrate spiritual and sexual intimacy fosters a state of wholeness, allowing us to deepen our relationships while nurturing our own inner growth.

One of the foundational practices for cultivating spiritual sexual intimacy is the art of mindfulness. Mindfulness invites us to be fully present, aware of each sensation and emotion without judgment. In a sexual context, this means savouring every touch, breath, and pause.

When we're mindful in intimacy, we're able to connect more deeply, creating a sacred space where both partners feel valued and understood. This practice encourages us to let go of preconceived notions and simply be present, reinforcing that every encounter is a unique expression of love.

Incorporating breathwork into intimate experiences can also elevate the spiritual dimension of sexuality. Conscious breathing helps align physical and emotional states, facilitating a deeper connection between partners. Techniques such as circular breathing or synchronised breathing between partners can create a rhythm that binds bodies and spirits together. By focusing on the breath, partners can enter a state of flow, transcending the physical and touching upon the divine.

Another practice that enhances spiritual sexual intimacy is the setting of intentions. Before engaging in intimate acts, partners may choose to share intentions or desires, infusing their experiences with purpose and direction. This can be as simple as wanting to feel more connected or as profound as seeking healing through shared vulnerability. By setting intentions, couples can use their intimacy as a vehicle for personal and relational growth.

Rituals play a significant role in deepening spiritual sexual connection. Rituals could be as simple as lighting candles, meditating together, or creating a sacred space free from distraction. These rituals become symbols of the commitment to each other and the shared journey of exploration. The gentle glow of candles or the soothing scent of incense can elevate the experience, marking it as special and outside of the ordinary flow of daily life.

Furthermore, Tantric practices invite individuals to experience sexuality as an extension of spiritual growth. Rooted in ancient traditions, Tantra offers exercises that help partners explore the dance of energy within and between them. This could involve practices such as chanting, eye-gazing, or exchanging light touch, all designed to awaken the senses and heighten awareness. Tantra teaches that sexual energy is a life force that can transform the mundane into the sacred.

Communication is a vital component of any spiritual sexual practice. Open dialogue about likes, dislikes, and boundaries fosters trust and mutual respect. Spiritual intimacy thrives in environments where both partners feel safe to explore and express themselves without fear of judgment. This kind of communication nurtures a bond that's not only physical but emotional and spiritual, reinforcing the deep commitments partners make to one another.

Exploring sexuality in a spiritual context also means embracing solitude and self-reflection. It's important to connect with one's own desires, fantasies, and limitations. Self-reflection can involve journaling about experiences, meditating on feelings that arise during intimacy, or simply spending time understanding one's own body. In doing so, individuals can approach their partners with a clarity and authenticity that enhances shared experiences.

The practice of touch as a spiritual sexual experience cannot be overlooked. Touch is a language that transcends words, capable of communicating love, care, and presence. Intentional, loving touch can dissolve barriers and foster a sense of unity. Whether through massage, caressing, or simply holding one another, touch becomes a pilgrimage towards deeper connection.

Spiritual sexual intimacy also involves relinquishing control, surrendering to the flow of the moment. This doesn't imply a loss of agency but rather a willing embrace of vulnerability. It's about allowing one's authentic self to be exposed and seen. In a spiritual sense, such surrender can lead to a form of transcendence, where individuals move beyond ego and experience a union that is transformative.

Integrating spiritual practices into sexual intimacy is an ongoing journey. Each partner must remain open to evolving individually while concurrently nurturing the shared connection. This journey isn't about achieving perfection but rather about embracing growth, learning, and the ebb and flow of life together. As partners engage in these practices, they may find that their sexual relationship becomes a sanctuary, a space where they can discover new depths both within and between themselves.

To summarise, the journey towards spiritual sexual intimacy requires intention, mindfulness, and an openness to explore deeper aspects of connection. By embracing practices like breathwork, ritual, and communication, individuals can transform their sexual experiences into sacred acts of love and unity. In doing so, they awaken to the profound interconnection of their spiritual and sexual selves, leading to a fuller, more balanced life.

Chapter 16:
Creating a Pleasure-positive Mindset

Embracing a pleasure-positive mindset is about reshaping the way we perceive pleasure not as a guilty indulgence, but as a natural and essential part of our well-being. It begins with recognising that sexual health is a vital component of our overall health, influencing not just our physical state, but also our emotional and mental landscapes. By challenging social taboos and personal insecurities that often cloud our judgement, we can nurture a space where pleasure is celebrated for its role in personal growth and connection. Cultivating a positive view towards sexual pleasure allows us to explore our desires without shame, fostering an environment where intimacy can flourish. It's about shifting perspectives and understanding that valuing pleasure enriches our lives, nurturing healthier relationships and a more profound sense of self. This transformative approach encourages us to question outdated beliefs, embrace open conversations, and ultimately integrate this positive outlook into every aspect of life, creating a balanced and fulfilling existence.

Shifting Perspectives on Pleasure

When we start talking about the concept of pleasure, particularly in the realm of sexuality, our thoughts are often clouded by a mix of cultural impediments, historical biases, and personal experiences. Yet, an exploration into shifting perspectives on pleasure reveals a myriad of benefits for our overall well-being. Rethinking pleasure, embracing its positive attributes, and dismantling old misconceptions is a transformative journey—a journey with the potential to enrich not only our sexual lives but every facet of our existence.

As individuals, we're influenced significantly by the cultural narratives around pleasure, many of which have depicted it as something frivolous or even sinful. These deep-seated beliefs can unconsciously dictate our attitudes and decisions, leaving us feeling conflicted and even guilty about seeking pleasure. But by altering our perceptions, we can break free from these constraints and move towards a more holistic acceptance of pleasure. This shift not only fosters personal growth but also enhances how we relate to others.

In the realm of sexuality, pleasure is often narrowly defined or misunderstood. The traditional views can be limiting, framing it purely around specific acts or outcomes rather than the broader, more intuitive experiences it can encompass. Redefining pleasure as a multifaceted experience allows us to consider the emotional, intellectual, and spiritual dimensions alongside the physical. Such a shift enriches our perspective, promoting not just a hedonistic pursuit but a balanced and integrated approach to pleasure.

It's crucial to acknowledge how diverse the experiences of pleasure can be. What brings joy and satisfaction can vary widely from one person to another. This variability is not only natural but is the essence of the human experience. By appreciating this diversity, we empower ourselves to seek and embrace different expressions of pleasure, whether they be through intimacy, creativity, connection, or solitude. Recognising these differences fosters a more inclusive and compassionate understanding of pleasure, turning it into a powerful tool for connection rather than division.

Psychologically, pleasure holds immense power. It is a motivator, a stress-reliever, and a significant contributor to mental health. The shift in perspective comes from acknowledging its role and allowing it to be a positive force in our lives rather than something to be controlled or suppressed. Building a mindset that recognises the importance of pleasure as a fundamental human need can help mitigate feelings of anxiety and depression, while enhancing both self-esteem and life satisfaction.

Moreover, the physiological benefits of embracing pleasure are significant. Pleasure activates certain neurotransmitters in the brain, such as dopamine and serotonin, which contribute to feelings of happiness and well-being. It's about leveraging this natural, biochemical response to improve our physical health, which in turn can enhance sexual vitality and increase longevity. Shifting our perspective to see sexual pleasure as a means of boosting overall health allows us to seek it not just for its own sake, but as an integral component of a healthy lifestyle.

The journey toward accepting a pleasure-positive mindset begins with introspection and education. It's about understanding where our current attitudes come from and challenging those that no longer serve us. This process often involves revisiting past experiences, examining the influence of culture and media, and being open to new information and perspectives. From this understanding, we can then begin to form new narratives that serve our true selves and enhance our well-being.

Central to shifting perspectives is the practice of mindfulness. By being more present and engaged in our bodies' sensations, we cultivate a deeper awareness and appreciation for the pleasures they can offer. It's about listening to what our bodies are telling us and responding with kindness and curiosity. This approach fosters a deeper connection with our bodies, enhancing pleasure while also promoting emotional and physical well-being.

Changing perspectives on pleasure is also about communication. With partners, this involves discussing and exploring what pleasure means within the context of the relationship. Open dialogues about preferences, desires, and boundaries not only enhance intimacy but also align the relationship goals with individual needs. Creating a safe space for these conversations is crucial for fostering a pleasure-positive mindset within relationships, reducing potential misunderstandings, and building stronger emotional connections.

In considering these shifts, it's important to remember the role of self-care and self-love. Accepting that each individual deserves pleasure is an act of compassion toward oneself. This means allowing oneself the time to explore what brings joy and satisfaction without judgement or pressure. Self-compassion in this context is crucial, as it helps dismantle any shame or guilt associated with prioritising pleasure in one's life.

Finally, supporting others in their journey toward a pleasure-positive mindset can extend our personal transformation into a broader societal impact. Encouraging education, dialogue, and understanding in communities can help demystify pleasure and promote a more inclusive and empathetic society. As we collectively embrace pleasure as a valued aspect of well-being, we open the door to healthier, more fulfilled lives for everyone involved.

As we navigate our unique paths, it's essential to recognise pleasure's vital role in our emotional and physical health. The simple act of shifting our perspective to see pleasure as a positive, nourishing force can have transformative effects, lighting the way to a more balanced and fulfilling life.

Cultivating a Positive Sexual Outlook

Cultivating a positive sexual outlook is a transformative journey that goes beyond mere sexual activity; it's about embracing and integrating sexuality as a core part of one's well-being. This perspective encourages individuals to adopt an open and affirming attitude towards their own sexual desires, experiences, and identities. It's a shift from viewing sexuality as a series of acts to understanding it as a rich and diverse part of the human experience.

At the heart of cultivating this outlook lies the concept of self-awareness. Developing a positive sexual mindset starts with recognising and reflecting on your own sexual beliefs and attitudes. Are these beliefs helping or hindering your well-being? Often, individuals carry societal or cultural misconceptions that can negatively impact their view of sexuality. By challenging these norms and narratives, you pave the way for a more liberated and personalised sexual outlook.

Central to this transformation is open-mindedness. Embracing an attitude of curiosity allows for exploration without judgment. It's about allowing yourself to learn from experiences, draw inspiration from diverse perspectives, and be willing to grow. In practice, this could mean reading about different sexual cultures, engaging in discussions, or experimenting with new facets of your sexuality in a safe and consensual manner. Each step you take towards understanding enriches your sexual perspective.

Everyone's sexual journey is unique, so it's essential to foster an environment of acceptance and patience within yourself. Embracing your own sexual identity and preferences can take time and may require unlearning prejudices that have been internalised over years. This process calls for patience and self-compassion. Remind yourself that it's okay to question, to take small steps, and to sometimes feel uncertain. Every moment of introspection brings you closer to a more profound and fulfilling acceptance of your own sexual self.

A positive sexual outlook also involves recognising the intrinsic link between mind and body. Your mental and physical states are intricately connected, and when they align, they enhance your capacity to experience pleasure. Practices such as mindfulness and meditation can be instrumental in this. They heighten body awareness and help you become more attuned to the sensations and emotions that accompany sexual experiences, thereby deepening your appreciation and enjoyment of them.

Moreover, understanding the dynamics of sexual energy is crucial for a pleasure-positive mindset. Sexual energy isn't confined to just physical interaction; it's an essential life force that can be channelled into various aspects of life, from creativity to emotional bonding. By nurturing this energy through conscious practices, you energise other dimensions of your existence as well, fostering overall well-being.

A supportive environment, where open dialogue about sexual wellbeing is encouraged, significantly bolsters a positive sexual outlook. This means being surrounded by individuals or communities that respect and nurture this growth. Engage with communities that value and uphold principles of respect, consent, and acceptance. Sharing experiences and insights with like-minded individuals can be incredibly empowering, providing a sense of belonging and validation on your journey.

Communication remains a pivotal aspect of cultivating a positive sexual outlook. Whether it's with a partner or oneself, being able to express desires, boundaries, and needs clearly and compassionately enhances sexual experiences. This form of communication requires vulnerability and honesty, but it ultimately leads to deeper connections and more fulfilling experiences.

Reflecting on role models and mentors can also shape a positive sexual view. Seek out figures whose relationship with sexuality embodies the values you aspire to integrate. This isn't to imitate them but rather to draw inspiration and courage from their experiences and journeys. Every story shared is a reminder of the diverse possibilities that a positive sexual outlook can offer.

It's important to acknowledge that external influences, such as societal and cultural forces, can impact sexual outlook. Media representations and cultural narratives can often perpetuate stereotypes or misconceptions. Remaining critical of these influences and actively seeking to educate oneself can help maintain a clear and empowering perspective on sexuality.

Ultimately, cultivating a positive sexual outlook is a continuous process that evolves alongside personal growth and life experiences. It's not about reaching a definitive state but embracing a mindset that is flexible, open, and grounded in self-affirmation. Each step taken towards this positive outlook nurtures your overall well-being, creating a harmonious balance between your sexual health and other facets of life. The journey, filled with self-discovery and empowerment, leads to a more fulfilling and enriched existence.

Chapter 17:
The Role of Sleep in Sexual Health

Sleep, often underrated, is a cornerstone of sexual health that ties into every facet of our intimate lives. When we slip into those restful hours, our bodies don't just recharge; they also regulate vital hormones that fuel desire, impacting both libido and performance. Like the gentle dance of night and day, the rhythm of sleep harmonises our physical and emotional states, creating a fertile ground for intimacy to flourish. A night of restorative slumber is akin to a well of vitality from which our energy springs, enhancing not only our physical capabilities but also our emotional connections. By prioritising sleep, we dive into a cycle of rejuvenation, where improved mood and cognitive function light the path to a more satisfying sexual experience. In recognising sleep as an ally, we're not simply treating symptoms of low desire or performance issues but fostering a proactive environment where sexual health can thrive. So, embrace those first yawns of longing for rest as the body's call for balance, and let every night be a step towards deepened sexual fulfilment and overall well-being.

Sleep's Impact on Desire and Performance

As we delve deeper into the interplay between sleep and sexual health, it becomes increasingly clear that sleep is a cornerstone of our biological and psychological well-being. But more than that, it's a powerful regulator of our sexual desire and performance. In the hurried pace of modern life, sleep often falls to the wayside, leading us to overlook its profound influence on our intimate lives. There's an elegance in the biology of sleep that extends its impact far beyond mere rest, enveloping sexual health in its embrace. Without adequate and restful sleep, the body's intricate systems of desire and performance can falter, presenting challenges that ripple through relationships and individual self-worth.

When we talk about sexual desire, we aren't merely addressing a biological urge but encompassing a myriad of factors that dictate our readiness to engage and connect. This readiness is finely tuned by the quality of rest we receive. Sleep acts as a restorative agent, rejuvenating both mind and body, replenishing neurotransmitter reserves and hormonal levels that underlie sexual desire. A well-rested individual often finds themselves more emotionally resilient and attuned to their partner's needs, leading to richer intimate experiences.

Hormones, the body's chemical messengers, play a pivotal role in sexual function. Cortisol, the stress hormone, inversely affects sexual desire when elevated, and sleep is a natural antidote to high cortisol levels. Furthermore, during deep sleep stages, the body regulates the production of testosterone and oestrogen, which are crucial for sexual desire and performance across all genders. Disrupted sleep, characterised by frequent awakenings or insufficient deep sleep phases, hinders this hormonal regulation, potentially diminishing sexual drive and impairing sexual performance.

Consider the complex dance of sleep cycles, comprising REM (Rapid Eye Movement) and non-REM stages, each with its unique contribution to overall health. REM sleep, often referred to as paradoxical sleep, is vital for processing emotions and memories, significantly impacting psychological and emotional intimacy. Restorative non-REM sleep, on the other hand, is crucial for physical recovery and energy replenishment. Together, they orchestrate a balance that fuels both the body and mind, enhancing the desire and the ability to engage in and enjoy sexual activities.

Moreover, the neuroscience of sleep reveals fascinating insights into its role in cognitive and emotional functioning. Sleep deprivation has been linked to diminished executive function, reduced empathy, and increased irritability, all of which can negatively impact sexual performance and intimacy. Unsurprisingly, individuals experiencing chronic sleep disruption often report lower libido, highlighting how essential sleep is to maintaining a healthy and enthusiastic sexual life.

The interconnection between the brain and sleep illuminates how foundational rest is for lucid sexual cognition and engagement. Sleep fortifies the brain's neural pathways, improving mood stability, clarity of thought, and emotional regulation. These enhanced mental states translate into a greater ability to connect with partners on a deeper level, nurturing mutual desire and satisfaction.

In exploring sleep's impact on sexual health, it's crucial to acknowledge the societal pressures that often distort our relationship with rest. From the pervasive culture of overwork to the glorification of minimal sleep as a badge of honour, these forces create a perfect storm for neglecting sleep health. Yet, it's in the prioritisation of quality sleep that we unlock the potential for profound personal and relational growth.

Creating a sleep-friendly environment and establishing a consistent sleep routine are practical steps towards harnessing sleep's full benefits. Simple adjustments, such as reducing exposure to blue light before bed, setting a regular sleep schedule, and ensuring a comfortable sleep space, can significantly enhance both the quality and quantity of sleep. By prioritising rest, individuals can reclaim their energy, sharpen their focus, and heighten their readiness for intimate, meaningful encounters.

In contrast, the repercussion of disregarding sleep is a cycle of depletion where irritability, decreased libido, and suboptimal performance become familiar companions. Left unchecked, this cycle can strain relationships and diminish personal well-being. On the flip side, when we harness the power of restful sleep, we align with the rhythms that sustain our energy, cultivate our desires, and fortify our performance, transforming how we connect with ourselves and others.

Sleep is not merely a passive activity but a dynamic process that imbues our waking lives with vitality, passion, and clarity. Recognising the importance of sleep is not just about avoiding dysfunction but is instead about aspiring to our fullest potentials both mentally and sexually. As we embrace the restorative powers of sleep, the pathways to vibrant sexual health open up, guiding us towards fulfilling and connected experiences that enrich our lives.

It's time to shift the narrative, positioning sleep at the forefront of our health priorities, not just for the promise of sexual enhancement but for the holistic benefits it offers to the fabric of our lives. By doing so, we don't just strive for better sleep; we pave the way for a more harmonious and fulfilling existence where sexual health thrives as an integral part of our overall well-being.

Improving Sleep for Better Sexual Health

In today's fast-paced world, sleep often finds itself at the bottom of our priority list. However, when it comes to our sexual health, skimping on sleep is a bit like pouring sand into a well-oiled machine. Without enough sleep, the intricate dance of hormones and emotions that fuels sexual desire and performance can quickly go awry. Let's explore how improving our sleep can have a profound impact on our sexual well-being.

To begin with, sleep is the body's natural way of rejuvenating itself, and this extends far beyond physical recovery. It plays a crucial role in regulating hormones, which are fundamental to sexual health. During sleep, the body balances key hormones like testosterone, which is vital not just for men's libido but for women's too. A deficiency can lead to decreased sexual desire and even contribute to erectile dysfunction in men. By prioritising a good night's sleep, we can help ensure these hormones remain at optimal levels, sustaining our sexual vitality.

Furthermore, the relationship between sleep and mood is undeniable. Insufficient sleep contributes to irritability and stress, which can dampen our inclination towards intimacy. Emotional readiness is essential for sexual well-being, as feeling mentally and emotionally off-balance can lead to a lack of interest in sexual activities. By getting enough sleep, we promote a more stable mood, creating an emotional climate that is more conducive to desire and connection.

Interestingly, sleep quality might be just as important as sleep quantity. High-quality, restorative sleep is characterised by smooth transitions between the different stages of sleep, particularly into rapid eye movement (REM) sleep. REM is the stage crucial for emotional processing and stress reduction. If we're not spending enough time in this restorative phase, our bodies miss out on these psychological benefits, which in turn can affect our sexual lives.

Now, you might wonder, how does one improve sleep to reap these benefits for sexual health? A variety of practical strategies can aid in enhancing both the quality and quantity of sleep.

Create a Sleep-conducive Environment: The ideal setting is cool, quiet, and dark. Consider blackout curtains and earplugs if ambient light or noise is unavoidable.

Establish a Regular Sleep Routine: Going to bed and waking up at the same time each day helps regulate the body's internal clock.

This consistency fosters smoother transitions into and out of sleep stages.

Limit Blue Light Exposure: With the omnipresence of digital devices, our exposure to blue light has increased, which can suppress the production of the sleep hormone, melatonin. Limiting screen time before bed can help counteract this effect.

Mind Your Diet: Avoid heavy meals and caffeine close to bedtime. Instead, opt for a light snack if hunger strikes.

Engage in Regular Physical Activity: Exercise promotes better sleep quality and increases the time spent in deep sleep. However, try to avoid vigorous activity close to bedtime.

Yet it's essential to remember that while these techniques are generally helpful, sleep issues can sometimes be complex. Conditions like insomnia or sleep apnoea might require more targeted interventions from healthcare professionals.

Besides these practical tips, consider the multi-faceted approach to stress management, including techniques such as meditation or breathing exercises, as these can significantly improve sleep quality and, consequently, sexual health. High stress levels are one of the most significant disruptors of sleep, creating a vicious cycle that impacts both quality of rest and intimacy. By reducing stress, we create the mental space needed for relaxation and restful nights.

Moreover, fostering an environment of emotional intimacy and communication with a partner can also enhance your sleep. When partners are emotionally in tune, they can better support each other's sleep routines and mitigate stressors that may intrude into the bedroom, be it figuratively or literally.

Integrating these practices into daily life may seem daunting at first glance. But consider them not as solitary changes, but as components of a lifestyle shift—one that prioritises well-being as a pathway towards fulfilling sexual health. This holistic approach, attending to both physical and emotional aspects, echoes throughout the tapestry of life improvements, weaving richer, more satisfying relationships.

Finally, let's not underplay the role of patience. Sleep patterns can take time to adjust, just as it can take time to see changes in sexual vitality. However, perseverance will bring about a harmony that enhances not just your nights but your days, too. This subtle interplay between sleep and sexual health is not merely a bonus for your mind and body but a foundational aspect of holistic well-being.

Acknowledging the significance of sleep in relation to our sexual health empowers us. It reminds us that taking the time to rest is not a luxury, but a necessity. In embracing this, we take a profound step towards a more vibrant, fulfilling life, intertwining the strands of sleep, desire, and overall health into the robust fabric of our well-being.

Chapter 18:
Managing Stress for Better Sex

In the symphony of life, stress acts as a persistent, dissonant note, overshadowing the harmonious melody of sexual well-being. When life's pressures mount, the delicate appetite for intimacy often dwindles, creating distance in the very connections that should provide solace and renewal. The link between stress and diminished desire is as undeniable as the first chill in autumn air, making stress management not just a priority but a necessity for a vibrant sexual life. Embracing techniques like mindfulness meditation, deep breathing exercises, and gentle physical activity can soothe the frazzled nerves, unlocking the innate passion that stress often shackles. By transforming stress from an insidious intruder into a manageable aspect of life, individuals can rebalance their energy and rekindle the flames of intimacy, weaving a tapestry of connection that enriches both body and spirit.

The Effects of Stress on Desire

Stress can be an insidious thief, quietly siphoning off desire and leaving a once-vibrant sexual landscape barren and uninspired. Many people underestimate the link between stress and sexual health, often seeking solutions through a myriad of other means without addressing the stressors at play. Understanding how stress affects desire is crucial for reclaiming one's sexual vitality and overall well-being.

When stress strikes, the body's natural response is to enter a state of heightened alertness, commonly known as the "fight or flight" mode.

This biological reaction triggers a cascade of hormones such as adrenaline and cortisol, which prepare the body to combat an imminent threat. While this mechanism is beneficial in acute situations, chronic exposure to stress hormones can wreak havoc on the body's systems, not least among them, the intricate dance of sexual energy.

Intimate connections require a certain level of emotional and physical availability, both of which can be compromised under sustained stress. Cortisol, often dubbed the "stress hormone," not only interferes with libido but can also suppress testosterone levels in men and women, directly impacting sexual desire. Meanwhile, feelings of anxiety or overwhelm can distract the mind, rendering it difficult to focus on the pleasures of a partner or even one's own body's sensations.

Moreover, stress rarely affects individuals in isolation. Its ripple effects often extend to relationships, creating friction or misunderstandings. When stress becomes a third wheel in a relationship, couples might find themselves more prone to conflict or emotional distancing, further eroding intimacy and desire. Communication falters, and the shared moments of connection that once ignited passion may dwindle into routine or feel like a chore. While the effects of stress are undoubtedly multifaceted, they're not insurmountable.

The first step towards managing stress is recognising its presence and impact. Often, individuals are so accustomed to high-stress lifestyles that they become blind to its effects on their sexuality. By becoming vigilant about stressors in daily life — whether they're work-related, personal, or a combination thereof — one can begin to untangle the knots that stress weaves in the fabric of desire. This self-awareness is empowering, as it allows one to take proactive steps towards positive change.

Engaging in stress-reduction techniques can significantly enhance sexual desire and performance. Activities like mindfulness meditation, yoga, or simple deep-breathing exercises can help lower cortisol levels and bring a sense of calm that rekindles the flames of desire. Physical exercise is also invaluable, releasing endorphins that counteract the negative effects of stress hormones while simultaneously boosting mood and energy.

In some instances, especially where stress is overwhelming or deeply entrenched, professional guidance may be beneficial. Therapy or counselling can provide much-needed support in navigating stress and its impact on sexual health. A therapist can offer personalised strategies to manage stressors and improve communication with partners, fostering a strong relationship foundation that supports mutual desire and exploration.

Restorative practices, like prioritising adequate sleep, can't be overlooked either. Sleep allows the body to reset and repair, reducing stress hormone levels and restoring balance to our hormonal milieu. With better rest comes clarity, energy, and an increased capacity for desire, underscoring the necessity of a healthy sleep regimen for better sexual health.

An integral part of regaining desire involves a shift in mindset. Cultivating an attitude that embraces and celebrates sexuality as a fundamental aspect of well-being can be transformative. Instead of viewing it as a luxury or mere indulgence, recognise it as a vital component of overall health. This mindset not only reduces guilt or anxiety often associated with sexual expression but also invites curiosity and openness into one's sexual experiences.

Finally, community support can play a pivotal role in managing stress's impacts. Engaging with others who understand and validate one's experiences can be both comforting and enlightening. Whether through support groups, workshops, or even conversations with trusted friends, sharing stories and strategies can provide fresh perspectives and foster a sense of solidarity.

It's important to remember that while stress can dull desire, resilience and passion are innate human qualities. By embracing stress-reduction practices and fostering an environment of open communication and support, it is entirely possible to revive desire and experience sexuality as a full and enriching expression of well-being. In doing so, individuals and couples can claim a more balanced, fulfilling, and joyful life, where desire flourishes despite life's inevitable challenges.

Techniques for Stress Reduction

In the interconnected web of health and wellness, stress arguably stands as one of the most pervasive disruptors. Not only does it impact our emotional and mental states, but it also casts a long shadow over our sexual desires and performance. Recognising and addressing stress isn't just beneficial; it's essential for fostering a fulfilling sexual life. By integrating practical stress-reduction techniques into our daily routines, we can create a fertile ground where desire and intimacy flourish.

One effective approach to managing stress is introducing mindfulness practices. Mindfulness, at its core, is about staying present in the moment, tuning into our bodies, and acknowledging the thoughts and feelings that pass through us without judgement. By practicing mindfulness, we train ourselves to let go of distracting worries and focus on the sensations at hand. This heightened awareness not only reduces stress but significantly enhances sexual experiences by allowing us to be fully present with our partners.

Breathwork, a simple yet potent tool, is another stress-busting technique. By consciously controlling our breathing patterns, we can activate our body's relaxation response. Engaging in slow, deep breathing sends signals to our brain that everything is alright, calming our nervous system and reducing the physical effects of stress. This is especially useful during intimate moments when performance anxiety might otherwise rear its ugly head. Just a few minutes of focused breathing can pivot the experience from stress-plagued to harmonious.

Physical activity should not be underestimated when it comes to stress reduction. Regular exercise helps elevate your mood by boosting endorphins—your body's natural feel-good chemicals. When we work out, we're not just easing stress; we're radiating positivity and cultivating a body more attuned to sexual vitality. Whether it's a brisk walk in nature, a dance class, or a sweaty gym session, physical activity relieves tension while enhancing body confidence and awareness.

While physical exercises abound, mental exercises such as positive visualization can also transform your stress landscape. By envisioning yourself in comforting, successful scenarios, you effectively rewrite your relationship with stress. Imagining joyful and intimate moments can set the stage for those experiences to become reality. This practice can shift perspectives over time, reducing anticipatory anxieties that often accompany intimacy.

Another pillar in the architecture of stress reduction is engaging in creative outlets. Creative pursuit—be it painting, writing, music, or dance—opens avenues for expressing emotions and relieving pent-up stress. Immersing yourself in a creative task diverts your mind from worries and channels your energy into something productive and fulfilling. This organic stress release not only liberates you mentally but can also invigorate your sexual imagination, fostering a more varied and adventurous intimate life.

Connecting with nature often provides a sanctuary for those besieged by stress. Whether it's a walk in the park, a hike in the mountains, or simply sitting in a garden, these interactions offer us not just tranquillity but a deep, intuitive recharge. Nature invites us to exist outside the confines of our restless minds and immerse ourselves in its rhythm. For some, this connection can awaken primal desires, anchoring us in the natural world and our place within it.

Let's not forget the power of laughter and its exceptional ability to diffuse stress. Sharing lighthearted moments with friends or loved ones can have a profound impact on our overall mood and stress levels. Laughter releases endorphins, lowers cortisol levels, and enhances our emotional connections with others. Incorporating more humour into our lives can make us more resilient to stress's detrimental effects, ultimately leading to a more relaxed and pleasurable sexual existence.

The role of touch cannot be overemphasized in managing stress for better sex. Human touch has been known to reduce heart rate, lower blood pressure, and leave us feeling more relaxed. Whether it's through massage, cuddling, or other forms of affectionate contact, touch encourages the release of oxytocin, often referred to as the "love hormone". This fosters a sense of closeness and reduces stress, creating an inviting atmosphere for intimacy.

Additionally, establishing a supportive network of relationships can act as a bulwark against stress. Confiding in trusted individuals can offer perspective and diminish the feeling of being overwhelmed. A strong support system not only defends against the harmful impacts of stress but also provides reassurance and strength during challenging times. Healthy relationships rooted in communication can nurture both mental well-being and sexual fulfilment.

Finally, it's essential to embrace the practice of gratitude as a stress management tool. By actively recognizing the positives in our lives, we divert attention from anxieties to contentment. Daily gratitude practices, whether in journaling or verbal affirmations, can rewire our outlook on life, making us more resilient to stressors and open to joy. A heart steeped in gratitude tends to approach intimacy with more warmth and less inhibition.

These techniques for stress reduction are not exhaustive but provide a robust framework for nurturing our overall well-being. In the interplay between stress and sexuality, deliberate practices can transform potential barriers into opportunities for connection, thereby enriching our sexual lives. As we cultivate these habits, the rewards echo beyond the bedroom, offering a more balanced and harmonious life experience. Remember, managing stress is not about eliminating it but rather transforming it, thereby enhancing our capacity for pleasure and connection.

Chapter 19:
Innovative Therapies for Sexual Wellness

In the ever-evolving landscape of sexual wellness, innovative therapies are blazing a trail towards a more holistic understanding of this vital aspect of well-being. Pioneers in the field are offering alternative modalities that go beyond traditional approaches, integrating mind, body, and spirit in ways that honour individual needs and desires. From the use of cutting-edge technologies to the rediscovery of age-old wisdom, these therapies are reshaping the future of sexual care. They invite us to explore and embrace unconventional paths, like energy-focused practices or therapeutic touch therapies, which aim not only to enhance pleasure but to foster deeper connections with ourselves and partners. As we open our minds to these possibilities, a fulfilling, balanced life where sexual wellness is a celebrated and integrated component becomes not just a hope, but an attainable reality.

Exploring Alternative Therapies

In the quest for sexual wellness, many are turning to alternative therapies that promise to tap into the body's innate healing abilities. These therapies, often rooted in ancient traditions, are being re-evaluated and adapted to suit modern life. They offer paths for rediscovery, renewal, and sometimes, profound transformation.

Among the most intriguing of these therapies is acupuncture, an ancient Chinese practice that involves the strategic insertion of thin needles into the skin at specific points. Acupuncture is believed to release blocked energy, or qi, and restore balance within the body. For some, this practice has been found to alleviate stress and anxiety, which are known culprits of decreased sexual desire. By promoting relaxation and harmony within, acupuncture can indirectly enhance one's sexual experience. It's worth noting that while some find this method effective, individual results can vary significantly.

Herbal medicine also plays a key role among alternative therapies. With roots reaching back thousands of years, herbal remedies have been used to stimulate libido, increase endurance, and balance hormones. Popular herbs such as ginseng, maca, and tribulus have been touted for their aphrodisiac qualities. These natural substances are believed to work by increasing blood flow and potentially balancing hormone levels. While promising, it is crucial to consult healthcare professionals before incorporating new herbs into your routine to avoid adverse effects.

Another approach gaining attention is holistic psychotherapy, which focuses not only on mental well-being but also on its interconnectedness with sexual health. This therapy aims to unearth deep-seated psychological blocks that inhibit sexual expression and joy. By addressing issues such as body image and anxiety, holistic psychotherapy can pave the way for a more fulfilling sexual life. This therapy often includes elements of mindfulness and meditation, encouraging individuals to stay present in their sexual experiences rather than being overwhelmed by past traumas or future worries.

Furthermore, couples' massage therapy presents an unconventional yet effective avenue for enhancing intimacy. This therapy transcends the boundaries of traditional massage by involving both partners, fostering a deeper connection through touch. The tactile experience can help reduce tension and promote relaxation, creating a safe space for vulnerability and closeness. By learning to communicate through their hands, couples can foster a non-verbal connection that nourishes their relationship on multiple levels.

A particularly unique therapy is tantra, an ancient spiritual practice that weaves together meditation, breathing exercises, and ritual, designed to elevate sexual intimacy to a transcendent level. Tantra isn't solely about sexual gratification; it's about channeling sexual energy and experiencing a deeper connection with oneself and a partner. Through tantra, one learns to prolong the sensory experience, facilitating an exploration of desires and boundaries. This practice celebrates the union of love and consciousness, providing profound insight into the essence of being.

Similarly, sound healing offers an intriguing exploration into alternative therapies for sexual wellness. Using frequencies and vibrations, sound healing aims to bring about a state of balance and healing within the body. Instruments like singing bowls, gongs, and tuning forks are believed to harmonise the body's energy fields, leading to relaxation and peace. The soothing sounds can help to quieten the mind and release emotional blockages, laying the groundwork for increased receptivity to intimate experiences.

Art therapy could also serve as an innovative exploration for those seeking alternative routes to improve sexual health. By engaging in creative expression, individuals might uncover subconscious barriers and unlock desires otherwise left unspoken. Painting, sculpting, or drawing can become a medium to express emotions and experiences not easily shared verbally, opening doors to greater self-awareness and acceptance. This therapeutic process helps tap into emotional depths and communicate one's inner world more freely, potentially improving one's sexual narrative.

Moreover, the rise of virtual reality (VR) therapy presents a cutting-edge frontier for enhancing sexual health. This burgeoning technology can offer immersive experiences designed to combat anxiety and enhance endothelial function—crucial for sexual arousal and satisfaction. VR can create simulations to safely explore fantasies or practice social skills, cultivating confidence and easing performance pressures. While still under study, VR therapy holds potential as a valuable tool in the vast landscape of alternative sexual health therapies.

In exploring these therapies, the objective is not only to foster healing but also to nurture an environment where sexual health blooms as an integral part of overall well-being. It's important to approach these therapies with an open mind and an understanding that what works for one might not work for another. Personal empowerment comes from exploring these options, discovering what resonates with you, and integrating those that align with your vision of sexual wellness.

Empowered with these diverse tools, individuals can traverse the vast and sometimes tumultuous landscape of sexual health. By combining traditional wisdom with modern insights, alternative therapies offer myriad pathways to enrich lives, deepen connections, and ultimately create a more balanced and fulfilling existence. Embracing alternative therapies is a testament to the power and potential within everyone to achieve holistic sexual well-being.

The Future of Sexual Care

As we gaze into the future, sexual care emerges as a beacon of hope and excitement, poised to transform lives through innovative therapies and advancing understandings. The ever-evolving landscape of technology, coupled with a growing awareness of the complexity of human sexuality, promises a future where sexual wellness is both a fundamental right and a holistic approach to health. We'll explore the possibilities that lie ahead in this realm and the potential impacts of these advancements.

In recent years, the conversation around sexual health has expanded beyond the basics of reproduction and disease prevention. We're seeing a shift towards recognising sexual satisfaction and joy as essential components of overall well-being. This shift, spearheaded by cutting-edge research and practice, is setting the stage for a future where sexual care integrates seamlessly with other facets of health care, providing comprehensive support that is both preventative and curative.

A vital part of shaping the future of sexual care is destigmatising conversations around sexual health. As society becomes more open and accepting, individuals are starting to seek help without embarrassment or fear of judgment. This cultural shift is catalysing a more profound interest in therapies that don't just address sexual dysfunction, but also enhance sexual fulfilment and translate to improved quality of life.

One promising area of development is personalised sexual health care. Much like how personalised medicine tailors treatments to individual genetic makeup, personalised sexual health care considers the unique physical, emotional, and psychological characteristics of each person. By utilising advanced diagnostic tools, future therapies could predict responses to treatments, thereby maximising efficacy and reducing trial and error.

Innovation in technology is set to play a major role in shaping the future of sexual care. Emerging technologies such as virtual reality (VR) and artificial intelligence (AI) have the potential to revolutionise therapeutic practices. For instance, VR therapy could offer immersive experiences designed to reduce anxiety or enhance arousal. Meanwhile, AI could provide real-time feedback and recommendations based on user data, creating customised therapy plans that evolve with the user's needs.

In addition to technological advances, we can anticipate a rise in integrative and holistic approaches to sexual wellness. These approaches focus on the interconnectedness of physical, mental, and emotional health. Practices such as mindful meditation, yoga, and breathwork are being increasingly recognised for their capacity to improve sexual well-being. Such practices open pathways for deeper emotional intimacy and a richer sexual experience.

The integration of traditional practices with modern science also promises an expansive horizon for sexual care. Practices rooted in ancient wisdom, like acupuncture and herbal medicine, might find new life through scientific validation and refinement. These therapies could provide support for hormonal balance, stress reduction, and energy flow—all contributors to a satisfying sexual life.

The future of sexual care will undoubtedly see an expansion of access to information and support. Digital platforms and telehealth services are already breaking barriers, providing advice, therapy, and community support to people in remote or underserved areas. Such platforms will become more sophisticated, allowing for better interaction, confidentiality, and customisation of care.

Education will continue to play a pivotal role in the evolution of sexual care. A comprehensive, inclusive approach to sexual education from an early age can promote healthier relationships and a positive body image, dismantling myths and fostering an environment where questions and discussions are encouraged. Empowering individuals with knowledge is crucial for making informed choices and taking charge of one's sexual health.

While optimistic, the path toward a future of advanced sexual care isn't devoid of challenges. Ethical considerations and privacy concerns will need careful navigation, particularly as technology becomes more intertwined with personal data. Balancing innovation with the protection of individual rights will form the basis of ethical conversations in the field.

Simultaneously, the development of robust policy frameworks will be crucial to ensure equitable access to these advancements. Ensuring that developments in sexual health do not solely benefit the privileged few is essential for a just and inclusive approach. Equity in access will help bridge the gap between different demographics, fostering a society where sexual well-being is universally attainable.

Ultimately, the future of sexual care invites us to reconsider how we understand and approach sexuality itself. It encourages a connective view, seeing sexual health as part of a larger network that includes emotional, physical, and spiritual dimensions. This vision doesn't just promise more pleasurable sexual experiences, but also a more comprehensive understanding of what it means to be healthy and fulfilled as human beings.

In this rapidly evolving landscape, the possibilities seem boundless, and each advancement offers the chance to enhance not just our sexual wellness, but our entire approach to life and health. By embracing these changes and nurturing an open dialogue, we're paving the way towards a world where sexual wellness is celebrated and integrated into our everyday lives.

Chapter 20:
Embracing Change and Growth

In the realm of sexual well-being, the dance between change and growth is both inevitable and enriching. As life's various stages unfold, one discovers the ever-shifting nature of desires and the expansive potential for personal evolution through sexual exploration. By acknowledging these changes not as hindrances, but as opportunities, individuals empower themselves to welcome new perceptions and experiences that foster deep-seated growth. This embrace of change encourages the nurturing of flexibility and openness, unlocking a deeper understanding of oneself and one's connections with others. True empowerment arises from this journey of self-discovery and growth, where adapting to life's rhythm becomes a pathway to not just survive, but thrive, building a fulfilling life that intertwines sexuality with holistic well-being.

Adapting to Life Stages

As we journey through different stages of life, each phase brings its own challenges and growth opportunities. Adapting to these changes is essential not only for personal development but also for maintaining and enhancing overall well-being. Embracing change and growth involves recognising that our relationship with sexuality is dynamic and constantly evolving. Life transitions, whether they're rooted in age, relationships, or personal achievements, often require us to reassess how we perceive and express our sexual selves.

Our sexual health and identity aren't static; they fluctuate, adapting to the rhythms of our lives. During adolescence, for instance, the exploration of sexual identity and desires can seem overwhelming, yet it is a vital part of forming a cohesive self-understanding. This phase is characterised by curiosity and a thirst for adventure, paving the way for deeper exploration and understanding in adulthood. As we age, our emphasis shifts from mere curiosity to a more profound connection with partners, and even with ourselves.

Midlife often brings about another layer of complexity concerning sexual health. Career changes, family responsibilities, and the physical changes brought by ageing can alter our sexual desires and performance. Yet, it is precisely at this moment that many discover a renewed sense of sexual awakening. The weight of experience provides a clearer understanding of personal desires and boundaries, encouraging a richer, more nuanced sexual expression. By embracing our evolving desires, we can craft a fulfilling holistic experience that integrates sexual health with both mental and physical wellness.

Ageing and its impact on sexuality call for resilience and openness to change. Society often magnifies the challenges of ageing, focusing on loss rather than growth. Yet, many find this time ripe with new possibilities. Older adults frequently report feeling more confident in their sexual and intimate relationships. This stage welcomes an intentional pursuit of pleasure and intimacy, often overlooked in younger years. Accepting these transitions fosters not just a healthy outlook on ageing, but also a revitalised approach to sex and relationships.

Changing life stages bring with them alterations in intimate relationships as well. Whether it's entering a new partnership, transitioning to parenthood, or experiencing the end of a long-term relationship, the ability to adapt is crucial. Each shift presents an opportunity for couples and individuals to redefine and renegotiate their sexual and emotional connections. Communication plays a pivotal role in these adaptations, fostering intimacy and understanding through honest and open exchanges.

Moreover, adapting to life's stages involves acknowledging and addressing the physical changes that accompany them. Hormonal shifts during events like menopause or pregnancy can significantly impact sexual desire and function. Instead of viewing these changes as obstacles, understanding and working with them can enhance overall well-being. Regular physical activity, good nutrition, and mindfulness can aid in managing the physical symptoms associated with such transitions, helping maintain a satisfying sexual life.

Personal growth during life transitions also means reassessing one's sexual identity and desires. What once excited and engaged us may shift, opening the door to exploring new facets of our sexuality. This exploration is crucial for continued personal development and satisfaction. Embracing these changes with curiosity rather than apprehension can enrich our lives and contribute to a more profound connection with ourselves and others.

The journey through life's stages reminds us of the impermanence of both physical and emotional experiences. Every stage offers lessons in resilience and opportunities for reinvention. Allowing oneself to feel joy, passion, and curiosity at any age fosters a robust sense of sexual well-being that transcends the physical body. A lifelong commitment to adaptability, openness, and education ensures that sexual health remains an integral part of our overall sense of self and life satisfaction.

Ultimately, adapting to various life stages in terms of sexual health demands a fluid approach. It's about embracing change, welcoming growth, and feeling empowered in one's evolving sexual identity. This perspective not only enhances personal and intimate relationships but also contributes to a more comprehensive understanding of well-being. By staying attuned to the changes life brings, and by approaching them with an open heart and mind, we can enrich our journey towards a balanced and fulfilling life.

Personal Growth through Sexual Exploration

In the realm of self-discovery, sexual exploration serves as a vital pathway to understanding oneself more fully. It's a deeply personal journey, where the process of embracing one's desires and curiosities often leads to profound personal growth. This exploration, though intimate, can hold the key to unlocking new layers of confidence and self-awareness. It's not merely about the physical acts but also about understanding what those experiences mean on an emotional and psychological level.

Exploration can greatly expand one's worldview, challenging preconceived notions about sexuality that might have been shaped by cultural norms or personal upbringing. As individuals venture into this journey, they begin to dismantle barriers that have long impeded personal growth. Shedding these external restrictions allows for a deep introspection into desires, needs, and boundaries, which are crucial components in crafting a fulfilled and balanced life.

The process often begins with self-acceptance—a foundational step that empowers individuals to embrace their unique sexual identity without fear of judgment. By accepting themselves wholly, including their sexual selves, individuals open the door to richer and more meaningful experiences. It is through this acceptance that personal growth takes root, allowing the intertwined relationship between sexuality and personal evolution to flourish.

An essential aspect of sexual exploration is the examination and understanding of one's own desires. This means being open to exploring different facets of sexuality in ways that feel safe and comfortable. As personal understanding deepens, so too does the appreciation for the role that sexual health plays in overall well-being.

When individuals have the freedom to explore, they can better articulate their desires and expectations in relationships, leading to more satisfying connections with partners.

Emotional resilience often strengthens through sexual exploration. Encountering one's limits and moving beyond preconceived boundaries instills a sense of achievement and strength. Struggles with vulnerability can be revealing and transformative, creating space for growth in self-esteem and self-worth. This isn't just about sexual confidence but extends to other areas of life, impacting professional interactions and social relationships alike.

Moreover, the journey fosters a sense of curiosity and continuous learning. Sexual exploration is not a destination but an ongoing process of discovery and adaptation. Each new experience and interaction can offer insights that shape and refine individual perceptions of sexuality. This perpetual state of learning invites individuals to appraise their comfort zones, further propelling their journey towards personal growth.

Having open dialogues about sexual exploration with partners can significantly enhance personal development. These conversations encourage transparency and understanding, fostering an environment where individuals feel secure to express their sexual needs and desires. Such interactions can mend or strengthen relationships, ensuring sexual health remains a shared responsibility that supports both individual and joint growth.

Furthermore, engaging in sexual exploration may challenge and subsequently redefine an individual's notion of intimacy. By experimenting with different expressions of sexuality, people often find themselves reframing their understanding of intimate connections—leading to a richer, more nuanced comprehension of what it means to share oneself with another. This, in turn, nurtures a deeper empathy and appreciation for others' experiences and perspectives.

Seeking guidance from sex-positive communities and professional resources can offer invaluable support during this exploratory journey. Such avenues provide safe spaces for individuals to share experiences and gain insights. Exposure to diverse narratives and practices enhances understanding and acceptance, nurturing an overarching sense of community and belonging that contributes positively to personal growth.

Ultimately, sexual exploration requires courage and honesty. By embracing these principles, individuals can harvest the fruits of growth and change. It's an empowering process, where the act of exploring and understanding sexual identity becomes a conduit for broader self-improvement. As one continues to experience and reflect upon their sexual journey, personal insights emerge, cultivating a self-aware and complete individual who is attuned to their holistic well-being.

Thus, personal growth through sexual exploration is an enriching journey characterised by continuous evolution. It's the thoughtful navigation of desires, emotions, and relationships that cultivates a balanced approach to life. Embracing this path not only leads to healthier sexual experiences but also empowers individuals to live more fully—encouraging them to embrace every facet of who they are with pride and authenticity.

Chapter 21:
Establishing Boundaries in Sexual Relationships

In the intricate dance of sexual relationships, establishing boundaries stands as a pillar of mutual respect and personal empowerment. Understanding and setting these boundaries is crucial for ensuring that every sexual interaction is rooted in consent and mutual desire. A well-drawn boundary is not a wall but a gate that facilitates healthy expression and connection, guiding partners in exchanging desires with clarity and confidence. Recognising boundaries involves an introspective journey, where individuals learn to articulate what feels comfortable and safe, paving the path to more fulfilling experiences. This practice of setting limits not only safeguards emotional well-being but also enriches sexual encounters by fostering an environment of trust and openness. By actively engaging in conversations about boundaries, partners affirm each other's autonomy while nurturing a space where profound intimacy can flourish. Embracing this respectful exchange allows relationships to thrive, enhancing the balance between shared experience and personal needs, and ultimately contributing to holistic sexual health and overall well-being.

Recognising and Setting Boundaries

In the labyrinth of sexual relationships, boundaries act as the compass that directs where one's comfort begins and another's ends. A nuanced understanding of these boundaries isn't just about knowing what you don't want; it's about vividly articulating your desires and limits, both to yourself and to your partner. Having this awareness doesn't happen overnight. It requires introspection, learning from past interactions, and sometimes, even a little courage to say "no" without guilt.

Recognising boundaries is fundamentally linked to self-awareness. It starts with an inward journey where you identify your own values, needs, and limits. Think of it as mapping out your personal landscape, where boundaries define the spaces you're willing to explore and those you prefer not to. This exploration involves asking yourself questions like: What makes me feel safe? What ignites my passion? What are my absolute no-go zones? Each question brings clarity, and this clarity forms the basis of setting effective boundaries.

On the path to this recognition, it's important to reflect on past experiences to uncover patterns. Have there been moments where you didn't feel respected or valued? These experiences often leave breadcrumbs that lead to deeper understandings of what your boundaries should be. Consider journaling these encounters, noting how they made you feel and how setting clearer boundaries might have changed the scenario. Through these reflections, you craft a more comprehensive understanding of your personal limits.

Setting boundaries then becomes an act of self-respect and empowerment. It's about confidently expressing your needs and limitations without fear of judgment. When you communicate your boundaries clearly, you foster an environment where your partner can do the same. This mutual respect nourishes a deeper connection, where both parties feel heard and valued. Open and honest conversations encourage a shared understanding, paving the way for a healthier relationship dynamic.

Communicating boundaries isn't a one-off conversation; it's an ongoing dialogue. As relationships evolve, so too can your needs and boundaries. Encourage regular check-ins with your partner to discuss both of your evolving landscapes. This practice ensures that both parties remain aligned and that any new boundaries are acknowledged and respected. Through such dialogue, you build trust and solidarity, reinforcing the foundation of your relationship.

One common mistake is viewing boundaries as barriers. Contrary to such belief, they're not walls designed to keep others out. Rather, they're guidelines that ensure mutual respect and understanding. This perspective shift from seeing boundaries as restrictive to protective can truly transform how partners engage with each other. It's akin to laying down a path where both individuals can walk together confidently, knowing the way ahead is understood and respected.

There's immense power in saying "no". This simple word can often be laden with fear of causing disappointment or conflict. But learning to use "no" without hesitation can be liberating. It asserts your right to personal agency and asserts your boundaries with clarity. Remember, "no" doesn't signify a lack of care or affection; it simply means that specific request or behaviour isn't aligned with your comfort at present.

Consider the role of non-verbal cues in boundary setting. Body language, tone, and even the pauses in conversation can signal discomfort or hesitation. Be attuned to these cues not only in yourself but in your partner as well. Often, they're the subtle alarms alerting you to potential boundary infringements. Honing your ability to recognise and respond to these signals can prevent misunderstandings, enhancing mutual respect and empathy.

Encouraging your partner to recognise and set their own boundaries is equally vital. When both individuals actively engage in boundary recognition, it creates a balanced field where both feel empowered and valued. Prompt your partner to explore their own comfort zones, share their findings, and listen actively when they communicate their needs. This reciprocity ensures that the relationship is a collaborative construct, continuously strengthened by mutual understanding and respect.

Recognising and setting boundaries doesn't mean eliminating spontaneity or passion from your sexual relationship. Instead, it creates a secure space where both are more likely to flourish. Boundaries provide clarity, allowing both parties to explore freely within the parameters that ensure safety and mutual consent. With boundaries established, the moments of spontaneity become even more meaningful and cherished, as they happen with conscious consent and awareness.

When misunderstandings occur, consider them opportunities for growth rather than setbacks. Discuss openly what happened and how it made you both feel. Use these discussions to reinforce and adjust boundaries where necessary. These moments, though uncomfortable, contribute significantly to the maturation of your relationship, enhancing both emotional intimacy and mutual respect.

Boundary setting is also about resilience. It teaches you to stand firm in your needs and to respect your partner's. It encourages personal growth and nurtures the courage to prioritise your well-being. Through this empowerment, you're better equipped to navigate not just sexual relationships, but all interpersonal interactions with transparency and integrity.

Recognising and setting boundaries in sexual relationships is fundamentally about fostering an environment where both partners feel safe and valued. It's a journey of self-exploration, communication, and mutual respect, integral to a nurturing relationship. Embrace this journey with openness, recognising that each step taken towards defining and respecting boundaries enriches the tapestry of your relationship, making it more vibrant, fulfilling, and resilient.

Respect and Consent in Sexual Interactions

Respect and consent are the cornerstones of any healthy sexual relationship. They're not just about abiding by rules; they create a foundation of trust and mutual understanding, pivotal for personal well-being. When we're tuned into our partners' desires and limits as well as our own, we foster meaningful connections that nourish our emotional and physical health. Establishing a culture of respect and consent requires ongoing communication and an active commitment to valuing each other's boundaries.

Consent is more than a one-time check-in; it's an ongoing dialogue. This dialogue should involve clear and enthusiastic agreement from all parties before proceeding with any sexual activity. Being attentive to both verbal and non-verbal cues allows us to understand whether our partners are comfortable, willing, and eager to participate. Consent should be freely given, without pressure or manipulation, and it must be reversible at any moment. If one partner is showing hesitation or seems withdrawn, it's essential to halt the interaction and address these concerns.

The importance of understanding consent lies in its ability to prevent harm and ensure that all involved feel safe and respected. The practice of asking for consent should not be viewed as interruptive or cumbersome but rather as a key ingredient in creating a mutually pleasurable experience. By prioritising consent, we cultivate environments where both partners can express their desires and limits openly, leading to more fulfilling and harmonious relationships.

Respect is equally crucial in nurturing sexual relationships. It's about acknowledging and valuing your partner's needs, wishes, and autonomy. Respecting boundaries means honouring the limits set by others, even if they differ from your own. This might involve being receptive to changes, acknowledging past traumas, or addressing varying levels of comfort with different types of intimacy. It's vital to foster an environment where discussion about personal limits feels safe and welcome.

This atmosphere of respect and consent doesn't just apply to physical interactions but also to the language and discussions surrounding them. Posing questions rather than making assumptions can clarify expectations and desires. "Would you like to try...?" or "How do you feel about...?" are ways to start these conversations. Thoughtful communication transcends mere words; it's about showing genuine interest and compassion in understanding your partner's perspectives.

However, establishing respect and consent isn't just reactive; it needs pre-emptive effort. Prior to engaging in intimate situations, discussing and setting personal and mutual boundaries ensures that both partners feel secure in expressing themselves. These conversations don't have to be rigid or clinical; incorporating them naturally into ongoing dialogue can shift the focus towards mutual enjoyment rather than concerns of boundaries being overstepped.

The dynamics of consent and respect must adapt as relationships evolve. New experiences, changes in personal circumstances, or shifts in emotional landscapes necessitate revisiting and potentially revising previously established boundaries. Life's complexities mean our needs and capacities for intimacy may change over time, requiring open discussions and adjustments. Embracing this fluidity helps maintain respect and consent as living, adaptable principles that secure ongoing connection and satisfaction.

Acknowledging past experiences and personal histories is another aspect of nurturing environments founded on respect and consent. Understanding that a partner's previous experiences may influence their current boundaries is key. Being considerate and patient establishes trust and safety, which are essential for fostering intimacy and joy. It's crucial to approach these discussions with empathy, allowing room for healing and growth.

Misperceptions about consent and respect can hinder their implementation. Some may mistakenly view expressing boundaries as confrontational or fear that requesting consent may disrupt spontaneity. Yet, true spontaneity blossoms when both partners feel secure in their boundaries, liberated by the knowledge that their desires and limits are acknowledged and respected. Reframing the role of consent as an enhancer rather than a barrier to intimacy helps dismantle these misconceptions.

Challenging societal norms and stereotypes plays a role in reinforcing the principles of respect and consent. Cultural narratives that perpetuate unhealthy dynamics or marginalise individuals based on gender, orientation, or ability must be confronted and dismantled. Establishing relationships that respect individuality and autonomy contributes to the creation of healthier societal standards overall.

Ultimately, the journey towards mastering respect and consent in sexual interactions is continuous. It requires introspection, an open heart, and a commitment to evolve alongside our partners. It's about paying close attention, listening with patience, and acting with kindness. These elements, in turn, not only enrich sexual relationships but also enhance personal and relational satisfaction, promoting a well-integrated sense of well-being.

Chapter 22:
The Intersection of Technology and Sexuality

In a world increasingly intertwined with technology, the landscape of sexuality is evolving at an unprecedented pace. Driven by digital innovation, the way people connect, communicate, and explore desire finds new avenues that both enrich and complicate intimate relationships. On one hand, digital platforms offer an expansive playground for self-discovery, fostering connections across distances and cultures that were once unthinkable. This digital intimacy, however, requires a mindful approach to ensure that it complements rather than overshadows the physical realm of relationships. Balancing screen time with face-to-face moments is crucial for maintaining the depth and authenticity that technology sometimes lacks. As technology and sexuality converge, individuals are called to navigate this intersection thoughtfully, integrating the benefits of digital advancements with the enduring value of personal intimacy. This harmonious balance is not merely about moderation but about crafting a fulfilling life where technology fuels connection without compromising the emotional and physical bonds that form the essence of human sexuality.

The Impact of Digital Platforms on Desire

The advent of digital platforms has undeniably transformed how we perceive, engage with, and nurture desire. From dating apps that promise to find you a soulmate with the flick of a thumb to social media algorithms that curate content echoing our deepest longings, technology has woven itself into the fabric of contemporary sexual experiences. These platforms offer a vast landscape of possibilities, but as with all forms of rapid progress, they come with their own set of challenges and complexities.

One cannot overlook the role of dating apps in reshaping human connection and intimacy. With platforms like Tinder, Bumble, and Hinge at our fingertips, the search for a partner has become both exquisitely convenient and overwhelmingly abundant. The concept of infinite choice, while empowering, can paradoxically lead to a form of paralysis where the search for the 'perfect' match turns into an endless swipe. This phenomenon, often referred to as the 'paradox of choice,' can dampen genuine desire as individuals become entangled in a cycle of comparison, forever chasing a mirage of an ideal partner.

Moreover, social media has emerged as a double-edged sword in the realm of desire. Platforms like Instagram and TikTok, with their emphasis on visual allure, can ignite fantasies and stoke desire, yet they can just as easily breed dissatisfaction. The curated perfection of digital life can distort our expectations of reality, igniting a dangerous interplay between aspiration and inadequacy. This has led to a growing disconnect where individuals may feel their offline selves can't compete with their online personas, creating barriers to authentic intimacy.

It's also worth noting the impact of digital platforms on sexual identity and exploration. For many, the anonymity offered online becomes a sanctuary where they can explore aspects of their sexual identity without fear of judgment or stigma. Communities form around shared identities and desires, offering support and validation in ways that might not be available offline. This can be incredibly liberating and serve as a catalyst for personal growth and understanding.

However, the darker side of this digital world is ever-present. The rise of cyberbullying, revenge porn, and digital harassment pose significant risks to those exploring their identities online. The potential for abuse and exploitation is heightened when desire is mediated through screens, often revealing itself in violations of privacy and consent. These breaches can have severe repercussions on one's sense of safety and willingness to engage further.

Another intriguing facet of technology's influence on desire relates to the consumption of sexual content online. Pornography, now vastly accessible, is a controversial yet undeniably influential component of the digital era. With instant access to a myriad of fantasies, desires can be explored in an unprecedented manner. Yet, the ease of access also risks skewing perceptions of consensual encounters and realistic expectations within relationships. For some, dependency on such content can diminish real-world intimacy, fostering disconnection from partners.

Digital platforms have also heralded new forms of sexual expression through virtual reality (VR) and augmented reality (AR), providing thrilling yet complex avenues for desire. These technologies allow for immersive experiences that can heighten arousal and creativity. In simulated environments, individuals can experiment without limits, pushing boundaries and discovering novel sensations. Yet, as these technologies advance, ethical considerations regarding their use and their impact on real-world relationships become paramount.

To navigate this intricate digital landscape, balance becomes essential. While technology offers unprecedented opportunities for connection and exploration, it's crucial to establish boundaries that protect emotional intimacy and personal well-being. This means cultivating an awareness of how digital consumption affects one's desires and relationships, and being mindful of the potential for over-reliance on technology to meet emotional needs that are best nurtured through human interaction.

Moreover, fostering digital literacy can empower individuals to make informed choices about their online interactions and consumption of content. Understanding the algorithms at play and recognising the constructed nature of online personas can help mitigate the negative impacts of comparison and dissatisfaction. This knowledge enables individuals to appreciate the actual tapestry of human desire beyond the screen's glow, promoting a more rounded sense of fulfillment.

In essence, the integration of digital platforms into the domain of desire is not inherently detrimental or beneficial. Instead, it highlights the evolving nature of human sexuality and the need for adaptability. As technology continues to innovate and redefine boundaries, it's vital for individuals to remain grounded in their values, aspiring to harmonise virtual and tangible desires in a manner that enriches their sexual well-being.

Ultimately, the impact of digital platforms on desire boils down to the choices we make in engaging with these technologies. With conscious effort, awareness, and a commitment to integrating digital experiences with real-world intimacy, individuals can navigate this era with grace and find genuine connection amidst the infinite possibilities on offer. Embracing the digital age, with its myriad challenges and opportunities, allows for a richer exploration of desire, one that honours both technology's potential and humanity's profound need for connection.

Balancing Technology Use with Intimacy

In today's digital age, technology permeates every facet of our lives, from how we communicate to how we nurture personal relationships. This pervasive presence holds significant implications for our intimate lives and sexual health. As we embrace the conveniences and connections technology offers, it's crucial to understand how we can balance its use to maintain and even enhance intimacy.

In the quest for intimacy, technology can both aid and hinder. On one hand, digital platforms allow for constant communication, enabling partners separated by distance to remain connected. Sharing messages, images, and videos can foster a sense of closeness, even from afar. However, the flipside sees technology often monopolising our attention, reducing the quality of time spent face-to-face with our partners. The irony is stark—while technology connects, it can also isolate.

The challenge lies not in using technology but in how we use it. Prioritising quality interactions over quantity is key. For instance, setting aside specific times for unplugged connection, where devices are put away, encourages more meaningful interactions. It's about creating a tech-free bubble where partners can engage without the distraction of constant notifications.

Moreover, technology has redefined how sexual education and exploration occur. Online resources have made information about sexual health, preferences, and orientations more accessible. This democratization of knowledge can greatly enhance sexual satisfaction and understanding between partners. However, it also necessitates a critical approach to discerning reliable sources from misleading content. To truly benefit, one must critically engage with the material, rather than passively consuming it.

The role of technology in bedroom activities is another dimension worth exploring. Apps and devices designed to enhance sexual pleasure are becoming predominant. While innovative, they risk diverting attention from the fundamental aspect of intimacy—the emotional connection. There must be a mutual understanding that while tech can augment experiences, it's not a replacement for the nuanced dance of human interaction.

Thus, deliberate conversations about the use of technology in intimate settings become paramount. Couples must negotiate how and when to incorporate technology in ways that enrich rather than replace their shared experiences. This might mean agreeing on boundaries regarding device usage or experimenting with digital tools together to ensure any tech-aided experiences are consensual and enjoyable.

On a societal level, the rapid shift towards digital everything leaves little room for traditional romantic gestures, often seen as relics of the past. However, reinvesting in simple, non-digital expressions of love—leaving handwritten notes, scheduling surprise dates, or engaging in joint hobbies—can reinvigorate relationships. Such practices serve as antidotes to digital fatigue, grounding partners in the tangible world of touch and presence.

Technology also reshapes how we perceive relationships and social norms surrounding them. The availability of online dating apps has influenced dating cultures worldwide, altering how relationships are initiated and developed. While providing myriad opportunities to meet potential partners, it can also lead to superficial engagements, where swipes replace in-depth conversations. Understanding these dynamics is essential in cultivating genuine connections in the digital realm.

Equally important is recognising the impact of social media on self-perception and relationship satisfaction. Constant exposure to curated images and seemingly perfect relationships can breed unrealistic expectations and dissatisfaction. A mindful approach to social media, where consumption is tempered with a critical eye, helps maintain realistic perspectives on oneself and one's relationship.

In balancing technology, self-awareness and communication become the cornerstones. Couples benefit from openly discussing how technology affects their relationship and collaboratively deciding on strategies to mitigate any negative impacts. Whether that involves establishing tech-free times, spending intentional time together, or engaging in digital detoxes, the aim remains clear—to prioritise intimacy.

The intersection of technology and sexuality isn't devoid of pitfalls, but it brims with potential. When used thoughtfully, technology can indeed enhance intimacy, making relationships more fulfilling. It's about harnessing its power as a tool, rather than letting it dictate the dynamics of our connections.

Ultimately, balancing technology use with intimacy is an ongoing journey. As digital innovations continually evolve, so too must our approaches in integrating these changes into our relationships. It's a dynamic balance that requires reflection, communication, and a commitment to preserving the essence of closeness and connection. In this way, our experiences remain authentic and our bonds, truly intimate.

Chapter 23:
Enhancing Desire Through Creativity

Igniting passion and keeping the flames of desire alive in any relationship often calls for more than just the everyday routine— enter the invigorating force of creativity. Creativity when interwoven with desire acts as a conduit for exploring yet-unseen dimensions of intimacy and connection. Our minds, by their very nature, thrive on novelty, and introducing fresh experiences or perspectives can rejuvenate relationships that might otherwise become stagnant. Whether through artistic pursuits, innovative role play, or even just a shared adventure, adding creative expression allows couples to explore their deepest fantasies in a safe, stimulating environment. It's about cultivating a playful and curious mindset, where both partners feel liberated to express their identities and desires without fear of judgment. By transforming the mundane into the magical through creative engagement, we renew not only our sexual appetites but also strengthen the emotional and mental bonds integral to a fulfilling union. As we continue to weave creativity into our intimate lives, it becomes a tapestry of shared experiences that manifest in a richer, more passionate connection.

The Power of Creative Expression

Creative expression, at its core, offers a transformative power that can profoundly enhance desire, weaving the very fabric that connects our sexuality with our broader personal universe. Often, creativity is perceived merely as the realm of artists, musicians, or writers. However, its reach extends far beyond traditional fields, serving as a gateway to deeper emotional and physical connections. By embracing creative pursuits, we allow ourselves to tap into reservoirs of emotional depth, often lying dormant under societal expectations and personal inhibitions. It's in these uncharted territories that desire isn't just sparked but ignited into a sustaining flame.

Exploring creative expression as a tool for enhancing desire isn't about becoming an accomplished artist. Rather, it's about stepping into spaces that encourage open-ended expression and experimentation. When we engage creatively, we unlock aspects of ourselves that are not necessarily accessible through everyday routines. This engagement allows for a deeper exploration of personal and relational narratives, fostering a unique space where desire and passion can thrive. Consider dance: the body, moving to music, creates a dialogue between partners that communicates more than words ever could. This physical expression not only releases endorphins but also strengthens the emotional bonds between individuals.

Artistic activities such as painting or creative writing invite you to express internal feelings and desires in new, often surprising ways. Creating a visual or written narrative opens up communication channels between different facets of our identity, including our sensual selves. By translating complex emotions into tangible forms, we give them a voice—and in doing so, may confront unspoken desires or concerns that impede our sexual wellness. Rather than cognitive or linear processing, this form of expression often allows an intuitive and organic understanding to emerge, reframing our own desires amidst broader life experiences and connecting dots previously left scattered.

Moreover, creative expression fosters a state of flow that can be incredibly liberating. When in flow, there's a harmonious alignment of our mind and body, and self-consciousness often fades away. Within this flow state, inhibitions melt, welcoming spontaneous and genuine expressions of desire. The focus on the present moment allows for a fuller engagement with our own feelings and those of our partner. Creative expression, in this context, becomes not a task to complete but a journey or an unfolding that promotes an authentic embracement of desire.

The collaborative nature of some creative endeavours, such as theatre or collective art projects, offers a shared platform for exploring mutual desires or challenges in a non-threatening environment. Engaging in such group activities builds trust and strengthens bonds, not just through the act of creation itself but through the discussions and insights that arise during the process. This shared creative journey can lead to greater empathy and understanding, essential ingredients for building and deepening relationships and desire.

Then, there's music—a universal language that transcends cultural barriers and speaks directly to the soul. Whether participating in a drumming circle, playing an instrument, or simply dancing rhythmically with a partner, music offers a cathartic release. These activities enrich our emotional landscape, providing a path to connect with deeper desires and energy levels. Music can be used as a medium to explore moods and energies, shifting them towards spaces of openness and receptivity, which are often crucial for sexual desire to flourish.

Additionally, these creative expressions offer practice in embracing vulnerability—a key ingredient in maintaining healthy desire. Vulnerability allows us to be fully seen and understood, without the façade we often present to the world. Engaging in creative activities requires letting go of judgments and barriers, encouraging a sense of authenticity and acceptance. By nurturing this aspect of ourselves, we cultivate an environment where desire feeds on the openness and honesty that vulnerability necessitates.

While creative expression boosts individual desire, it also provides tangible benefits to relationships. By participating in shared creative experiments, partners can forge new narratives, developing a joint language that mirrors their evolving connection and understanding. These experiences, when shared, become pivotal moments—anchors that partners can return to when seeking connection or solace.

As creative expression fosters exploration and connection, it indirectly helps in dismantling blockages or societal constructs that might stand in the way of desire. Exploring diverse styles and modes of expression can be a practice of reclaiming autonomy over one's narrative, from which springs an invigorated sense of self and desire. It's in this empowerment that creative expression not only enhances desire but aligns it with personal growth and fuller self-acceptance.

Imagine crafting a poem together with a partner, inspired by the senses. Each word chosen and each stanza built is a testament to shared experiences and desires, captured in ink and imagination. Doing so not only affirms what is felt but builds a collaborative story—one that includes both the spoken and unspoken words of desire. These stories, crafted through creative expression, become vibrant parts of a couple's shared journey, nestled in their collective consciousness.

Finally, creative expression introduces an element of playfulness and curiosity into our lives. Whether it's trying a new form of art or exploring existing interests, the process can inject fun and spontaneity into routine experiences. This playfulness encourages risk-taking and experimentation, which are vital not just for creative projects but for keeping desire alive and dynamic.

In our intensely structured lives, the permission granted by creative expression to explore unfettered by convention is valuable beyond measure. The freedom to delve into differences, explore boundaries, and discover shared spaces is as essential to nurturing desire as it is invigorating to personal and collective health. Through creativity, we find pathways that entwine our emotional, mental, and sexual selves, leading to personal liberation and an unarguably richer tapestry of desire.

Strategies for Keeping Desire Alive

Desire, much like a living organism, needs nourishment and attention to thrive. Creativity plays a pivotal role in ensuring this aspect of our lives remains vibrant and fulfilling. It's about cultivating a space where curiosity, exploration, and romance can bloom. Whether it's through shared experiences or personal introspection, keeping the flame alive requires a dash of ingenuity and a willingness to embrace the unknown.

Begin by incorporating novelty into your intimate life. Humans are inherently curious creatures, and by engaging with new experiences together, you can keep desire both palpable and exciting. This doesn't mean that each interaction needs to be groundbreaking. Sometimes, it's the subtle shifts, like changing your daily routine or trying a new interest, that can rekindle passion. Imagine taking a dance class together, or simply cooking a meal you've never attempted before. The unpredictability and newness of these activities can reawaken latent desires and deepen your emotional connection.

Another key strategy is to harness the power of creative storytelling within the relationship. Picture the tales you weave as threads binding your shared world. By creating and recounting stories together—whether they're imaginary adventures or reflections on your journey as a couple—you build a canvas that is both intimate and ever-expanding. These stories can be as elaborate as crafting a fictional narrative about a dream holiday or as simple as sharing memories of your first meeting. This shared creativity can reinvigorate desire by reminding you of the bonds and experiences that make your relationship unique.

Engage with artistic mediums—music, painting, writing—as a way of expressing and exploring your desires. There's a profound connection between art and emotion, and by tapping into these forms of expression, you can access deeper levels of intimacy. You don't need to be an artist to benefit from this; even listening to a new genre of music or visiting an art gallery can evoke emotions and stimulate conversation that enriches your relationship. Art often speaks to the nuances of human experience, resonating on levels words alone cannot reach. This, in turn, cultivates a fertile ground for desire to flourish.

Reflecting on one's individual creativity can also feed into a richer shared experience. Encourage each other to explore personal projects or hobbies that ignite passion. When both partners are engaged in activities that inspire them, the energy and enthusiasm they bring back to the relationship are contagious. Sharing these creative escapades with your partner gives insight into each other's inner worlds, fostering a sense of closeness and respect for personal growth. This dual focus— on the self and the shared—keeps desire dynamic and nurtures a relationship that values both togetherness and individuality.

It's also crucial to continuously communicate your desires and boundaries creatively. Traditional conversations about needs and wants can sometimes be mundane, so why not infuse them with a bit of creativity? Write letters or keep a shared journal where both partners can freely express thoughts and feelings. This non-verbal form of communication can sometimes unveil desires that might be challenging to articulate in spoken form. Moreover, this practice can become a treasured ritual that strengthens emotional intimacy.

Introducing elements of playfulness can bring a refreshing lightness to your relationship. Laughter and fun are essential ingredients in the recipe for sustained desire. Whether through playful banter, engaging in light-hearted games, or embarking on spontaneous adventures, nurturing a spirit of play keeps the relationship from becoming overly serious. It creates a sense of joy and freedom, allowing both partners to shed their daily worries and reconnect on a more primal, pleasurable level.

Finally, don't underestimate the power of personal rejuvenation and self-care in keeping desire alive. Taking time for oneself—and encouraging one another to do the same—ensures that you both bring the best version of yourselves to the relationship. This means honouring your individual needs, be it through meditation, physical activity, or quiet reflection. A well-rested, fulfilled partner is far more capable of contributing to a healthy, vibrant relationship. When both partners take this responsibility seriously, desire is more likely to sustain itself naturally.

These strategies aren't about rigid schedules or checklists but rather embracing a mindset that values innovation and connection in equal measure. By breathing creativity into how we express and nurture desire, we not only keep it alive but invite it to grow in ways that are profoundly enriching. At its core, this approach encourages us to hold space for the mystery and magic that desire inherently possesses, allowing it to evolve with time and experience.

Chapter 24:
Building a Supportive
Sexual Community

Creating a supportive sexual community is all about finding allies in your journey toward sexual well-being and growth. It involves cultivating safe spaces where open dialogue flourishes, and shared experiences become a rich source of wisdom and strength. In such communities, individuals can explore their desires, confront societal norms, and celebrate the diversity of human sexuality. This shared journey contributes significantly to personal empowerment and collective understanding, offering participants a sense of belonging and encouragement. As you step into these spaces, the bonds formed not only enhance your personal sexual exploration but also enrich your overall well-being, demonstrating the profound impact that supportive networks can have on our lives. Embracing such a community inspires growth, builds resilience, and acknowledges that sexual health is a vital component of holistic wellness. By engaging collaboratively, we recognise that our journeys, while uniquely personal, are deeply interconnected, and through this unity, we can foster environments of acceptance, learning, and genuine connection.

Finding Allies in Sexual Exploration

Embarking on a journey of sexual exploration can be an exhilarating and transformative experience. It's a path towards self-discovery, empowerment, and a deeper understanding of one's desires and preferences. However, it's not a journey that needs to be travelled alone. Finding allies who share similar goals or experiences can provide invaluable support and encouragement. Building such connections can enrich your experience and offer a sense of community.

Once upon a time, conversations about sexual exploration were often hushed, relegated to whispered secrets shared in the privacy of close friendships or behind closed doors. Today, thanks to evolving social norms and the expanding landscape of digital communication, discussions about sexuality are becoming more open and inclusive. This shift has made it possible to find allies and build communities that can provide support and shared understanding.

So, why is finding allies crucial to sexual exploration? First and foremost, having allies offers emotional support. Exploring sexuality can bring up a range of emotions, from excitement to vulnerability. It's comforting to know that others have tread a similar path and can offer empathy, advice, or simply an understanding ear. Allies can validate your feelings and experiences, making you feel more confident in your journey.

Moreover, engaging with a community of allies can open doors to new perspectives. Everyone's sexual journey is unique, shaped by a myriad of factors like culture, upbringing, and personal experiences. By interacting with others, you gain insights into different viewpoints and experiences, broadening your own understanding of sexuality. This exchange of ideas can lead to greater personal growth and a more nuanced appreciation of sexual diversity.

Joining online forums or groups dedicated to sexual exploration is a great starting point. These spaces often facilitate discussions on various topics, from discovering sexual preferences to exploring kink or polyamory. They are often moderated environments where you can seek advice or share experiences without fear of judgment. You may find groups on social media platforms, dedicated online communities, or more private forums that ensure anonymity.

While online communities offer valuable opportunities for connection, in-person engagement shouldn't be overlooked. Local meetups, workshops, or discussion groups focused on sexual health and exploration can provide a more personal touch. Such gatherings often create a safe space for sharing, learning, and growing with others who are embarked on their own journeys of discovery. These real-life interactions can lead to the formation of genuine friendships and supportive networks.

Building allies in sexual exploration is not just about finding people who share your specific interests or kinks. It's also about engaging with those who support your right to explore and embrace your sexual identity in a way that feels authentic to you. These allies respect boundaries, prioritise consent, and champion sexual well-being.

Educational workshops and retreats centred on sexual wellness and exploration can also be profound opportunities for allyship. These immersive environments often bring together experts and novices alike, offering a blend of learning and partnership. During such events, you might connect with like-minded individuals and benefit from shared experiences that can enrich your understanding and practice.

Let's not forget the power of literature and media as allies in your exploration. Books, podcasts, and documentaries can serve as silent yet powerful allies, providing knowledge and sparking inspiration. They also introduce you to the broader community of thinkers, writers, and creators passionate about sexual exploration, connecting you in spirit and thought.

As you step into this multifaceted community, remember the importance of communication. Establishing open dialogue with your allies is crucial to ensure that all parties feel safe, respected, and heard. Whether you're discussing boundaries, sharing experiences, or engaging in discussions about sexual ethics, transparent communication fosters trust and mutual respect.

Furthermore, as you build this network, consider the role of intersectionality in your allies' journeys. Recognise that each individual's experience is shaped by numerous factors, including gender, race, orientation, and cultural background. By acknowledging these layers, you develop a deeper empathy and understanding, allowing for more meaningful connections.

A community that values diversity and inclusion becomes a fertile ground for both personal and collective growth. As allies, you have the opportunity to learn from one another's unique perspectives, which in turn enriches the overall exploration for everyone involved. It's about celebrating both commonalities and differences, recognising that there is no single "right" way to explore sexuality.

Finally, a crucial aspect of finding allies is to ensure that support is reciprocal. While it's important to receive encouragement and validation, offering the same support to others cultivates a healthy, balanced community. Being an ally to someone else can be just as rewarding and enlightening; it encourages empathy and fosters a deeper connection with your own experiences.

As you continue your journey, remember that finding allies is not a final destination but an evolving process. Your community may change as you grow, and that's perfectly okay. Each new ally can introduce you to new ideas, adventures, and possibilities, continually enriching your exploration.

In summary, finding allies in sexual exploration is a transformative endeavour that significantly enhances your journey. It provides emotional support, broadens perspectives, and fosters an inclusive community where diversity is celebrated. With the right allies, you can turn what might have been a solitary journey into a shared adventure, full of discovery, growth, and empowerment.

The Benefits of Community and Shared Experience

In a world where individualism is often celebrated, the power of community might sometimes get overlooked, especially in matters of sexuality and well-being. Engaging with a supportive sexual community can bring significant benefits that transcend personal growth and enhance overall quality of life. At the heart of it, shared experiences can foster a sense of connection and understanding that might otherwise be elusive.

One profound benefit of building a sexual community is the reduction of shame and stigma associated with sexual exploration and expression. When individuals gather to share their experiences and perspectives, it creates an environment where everyone feels more comfortable to express themselves openly. This openness helps dismantle the barriers of judgment and ridicule that often surround sexual discourse. People find solace in knowing they aren't alone in their feelings, fantasies, and challenges. This realisation can be a powerful catalyst for radiating self-acceptance and embracing one's sexual identity without fear.

Moreover, shared experiences within a community encourage learning and knowledge exchange. The diversity of backgrounds and experiences within a group creates a rich tapestry of information, insights, and advice. Whether it's learning about new techniques, understanding different sexual orientations, or even discovering ways to communicate more effectively with a partner, the pool of collective wisdom acts as a wellspring of resources. This knowledge expansion can lead to better health choices, more satisfying relationships, and ultimately, a deeper understanding of one's own needs and desires.

Emotional support is another cornerstone benefit of a sexual community. Many people face struggles that they might not be comfortable discussing even with close friends or partners. A supportive community offers a safe space for individuals to share their vulnerabilities, fears, and concerns. This emotional sharing not only unburdens individuals but also reinforces the communal bonds, creating an empathetic circle where members feel valued and understood. The comfort of knowing that others have gone through similar journeys and emerged stronger can be incredibly reassuring.

Inspiration and motivation are equally important outcomes of engaging with a community. Witnessing the courage and transformations of others can ignite a sense of possibility within oneself. Success stories, personal triumphs, and even tales of overcoming adversity can encourage individuals to step outside their comfort zones and explore new facets of their sexuality and passions. This motivational spark can lead to personal growth and open the door to more fulfilled and intentionally crafted sexual lives.

However, it's not solely about receiving benefits; being part of a community also involves contributing to the shared experience. This reciprocal exchange enhances one's sense of purpose and belonging. When individuals share their stories, insights, and support, they not only help others but also solidify their own understanding and appreciation of their sexual self. Such contributions nurture an environment of mutual growth and enrichment, leading to stronger interpersonal connections and a more cohesive community.

Additionally, the social dimension of a sexual community can't be underestimated. Beyond the more serious aspects, communities provide a space for joy, celebration, and expression. Events, workshops, and social gatherings offer opportunities to connect with like-minded individuals in a relaxed setting. These interactions often lead to lasting friendships and, in some cases, partnerships based on a deep and genuine understanding of one another's desires and journeys.

From a broader perspective, sexual communities also play a pivotal role in social change. By elevating conversations around sexual well-being and rights, they challenge societal norms and push for more inclusive and accepting cultures. These groups act as champions of change, advocating for policies and practices that respect and support diverse sexualities and identities. Being part of such a community means contributing to a movement that's bigger than oneself, and standing alongside others to pave the way for future generations.

While each individual's journey to sexual well-being is unique, the advantages of engaging with a community and sharing in their collective experience are universal. From empowering personal growth to driving societal change, the benefits intersect and influence myriad aspects of life. As more people connect and share their sexual journeys, the ripples of understanding, respect, and acceptance continue to expand, enriching not only individual lives but the wider world as well. Embracing community transforms what might be a solitary journey into a shared adventure of exploration, understanding, and empowerment.

Chapter 25:
Achieving Sexual Synergy

In the quest to achieve sexual synergy, we enter a transformative space where health and desire harmoniously intertwine, lifting each area of one's life to new heights. It's about cultivating an awareness that sexual health isn't just a sidebar to wellness—it's a vital thread, weaving through the fabric of our entire being. By integrating practices that enhance sexual vitality into daily routines, balancing physical, emotional, and mental well-being becomes attainable. Consider how fostering a nuanced understanding of your own needs and those of your partner can deepen intimacy, creating a positive feedback loop for both health and desire. Embodying sexual synergy is not about perfection but embracing a conscious evolution towards fulfilling relationships that celebrate mutual energy and connection, leading us to a more vibrant, well-rounded life.

Integrating Sexual Health into Daily Life

Integrating sexual health into one's daily life isn't just about enhancing intimacy; it's about embracing an enriching and holistic approach to well-being. Sexual health impacts physical fitness, mental serenity, and emotional balance. To appreciate its full potential, consider it a vital component much like nutrition or exercise. It's not a separate entity but rather interwoven into the fabric of daily existence, impacting all sphere of life.

Each day presents an opportunity to incorporate practices that nurture sexual health. This doesn't necessarily mean a singular focus on sexual acts but rather fostering an environment where words, gestures, and introspections cultivate a heightened awareness of oneself and one's partner. By embedding these practices, we naturally enhance our self-awareness and relationships.

Begin with simple yet powerful habits. Much like any beneficial routine, consistency proves key. Mindful breathing or a short meditation session can open channels to sexual energy, allowing it to flow more freely through us. These practices lower stress, clear mental blockages, and set the stage for a more profound connection between body and mind.

Connections don't always have to be solely verbal; intentional touch can be transformative too. Simple, thoughtful contact like a gentle hand on a partner's back or a shared moment of eye contact builds emotional bridges, fostering intimacy and sexual synergy without needing words. These are the understated ways in which daily life can become a canvas for sexual health exploration.

Beyond touch, consider your interactions with your environment. A morning yoga session, for instance, can awaken more than just muscles. Paired with deliberate breathing, yoga stretches the boundaries of what we thought possible, rejuvenating both body and spirit. Its impact often extends into the day, crafting an open, receptive mindset toward intimacy.

The role of communication in developing sexual synergy can't be overstated. Yet, more than just discussing desires, it's about active listening and creating a space where both parties feel safe and respected. Open dialogue enables partners to express themselves freely, leading to a deeper understanding of collective needs and aspirations.

Your diet also plays an integral role in how sexual health manifests daily. Embracing a nutrient-rich diet influences more than just physical vitality; it kindles your body's natural energy reserves. Foods laden with essential vitamins and minerals boost libido, reinforce stamina, and better the overall mood, paving the way for vibrant sexual health.

While food fuels your internal engine, staying physically active keeps it running smoothly. Exercise acts as an invigorating force, boosting blood flow and releasing endorphins that heighten sexual pleasure. It's a natural method to bolster both physical and mental attunement, fostering a sense of readiness for intimate moments.

Equally crucial is the understanding that achieving synergy requires mental clarity. Practice identifying and managing stressors that could hinder your sexual well-being. Whether through mindfulness or structured relaxation techniques, incorporating stress-reduction practices into your daily routine maintains a balance between productivity and the nurturing of sexual energy.

Explore techniques that harness creativity to fuel desire. This could be through art, writing, or simply engaging in playful ventures with a partner. Creative expression finds a way to bypass conventional barriers, rekindling passion and reinvigorating connections. Remember, a spontaneous dance or doodle shared with a loved one can often say more than any conversation.

Respect and boundaries form an essential foundation for integrating sexual health throughout life. It's vital to always consider consent and ensure that all interactions are built on mutual respect and enjoyment. Understanding and establishing boundaries allows each individual to feel secure and valued, fostering a healthy environment for intimacy to flourish.

Lastly, acknowledge that technology will play its part in modern integrations of sexual health. Whether it's setting digital boundaries to enhance real-world connections or utilising apps for health tracking and communication, technology can be a powerful ally or a disruptive force, depending on its application. Balance is the key to reaping its benefits while nurturing authentic interactions.

The pursuit of sexual synergy is ongoing, an evolving dance where those involved adjust to the rhythms of life. By integrating sexual health into daily practice, people don't just strive for better intimacy but also experience growth in personal well-being. Each decision made consciously contributes to a life enriched by the profound harmony between health and desire.

Creating a Harmonious Balance Between Health and Desire

The quest for a balanced integration of health and desire is one that many embark upon, yet few truly master. This delicate balance is essential for achieving sexual synergy, where both wellbeing and passion coexist in seamless harmony. It requires a keen understanding of what fuels desire while maintaining a commitment to overall health.

At the heart of this integration lies self-awareness. Staying attuned to our body's cues and recognising the ebb and flow of desire can lead to deeper insights into our physical and emotional health. Understanding what drives our sexual desire allows us to address the varying needs of our body and mind. Often, an imbalance occurs because desires are either suppressed or pursued without considering their broader impacts on our health, leading to frustration and disharmony.

One of the first steps in creating this harmony involves prioritising mental clarity and emotional peace. Many of us underestimate the power of stress and psychological blocks in dampening our desire. When stress levels are high, the body's natural inclination is to focus on survival, not passion. Techniques such as mindfulness, meditation, and gentle physical exercise can help alleviate mental clutter, opening pathways to both relaxation and desire.

Nutrition also plays a pivotal role in balancing health and desire. The foods we consume can directly impact our libido, energy levels, and overall wellbeing. An imbalance in nutrition can lead to a lack of vitality, which subsequently affects sexual desire. Consuming a well-rounded diet rich in nutrients not only benefits physical health but also enhances sexual energy, making for a more harmonious relationship between health and desire.

Physical fitness shouldn't be overlooked when we talk about achieving a harmonious balance. Regular exercise boosts mood and energy levels, and it's also beneficial for sexual health. Activities like yoga not only strengthen the body but also promote flexibility, increase blood flow, and help reduce stress, which in turn fuels desire. Exercise can be a powerful tool that bridges the gap between physical health and sexual vitality.

Open, honest communication with one's partner is crucial in maintaining harmony. Verbalising desires and health concerns is often difficult, yet it plays an essential role in mutual understanding and compassion. Effective communication strategies can help partners align their health goals with their intimate desires, creating a path for collaborative growth and mutual satisfaction.

Hormonal balance further influences this dynamic harmony. Understanding how hormones interplay with desire and health can empower individuals to make informed choices regarding lifestyle and diet. Natural methods of balancing hormones, such as proper sleep hygiene, nutrition, and stress management, support both vitality and sexual well-being, contributing to a holistic balance.

The landscape of sexual identity and expression is vast and diverse, and exploring one's sexual self can be liberating. Embracing individual sexual identities while being attuned to one's health disciplines can significantly augment this harmonious balance. Such acceptance allows for alignment of desires and health priorities, fostering a deeper connection with oneself and with partners.

The ageing process introduces another facet to consider in achieving balance. As the body changes, so do the expressions and experiences of sexual desire. Awareness and adaptation to these natural changes, coupled with lifestyle modifications, can maintain a vibrant expression of sexuality throughout the lifespan. Viewing ageing as an opportunity to deepen and redefine intimacy can enhance the synergy between health and desire.

Creating a harmonious balance between health and desire also involves overcoming sexual dysfunction. Many may face physical or psychological barriers that hinder their intimate lives, but addressing these with compassion and understanding is key. Exploring various solutions and remaining open to different therapies can help heal these aspects, allowing for a healthier expression of desire without compromising overall well-being.

Ultimately, cultivating a pleasure-positive mindset is crucial. Shifting perspectives on what pleasure means and how it integrates into our lives supports a more balanced approach to sexuality. Encouraging positive sexual attitudes and embracing the joys of intimacy without guilt or shame pave the way for authentic and fulfilling expressions of desire that align beautifully with health goals.

In sum, achieving sexual synergy requires a deliberate effort to synthesise desire with health. It involves recognising the interconnectedness of body, mind, and emotions, all while nurturing open dialogues and embracing changes with grace. By focusing on this balance, individuals can experience more satisfying relationships and a greater sense of personal well-being.

Conclusion

The journey through this book has traversed a landscape often uncharted yet innately familiar. Sexual health, a fundamental aspect of human existence, intertwines with every facet of our lives—from our mental and physical health to our emotional and social connections. Throughout the chapters, specific threads have illuminated the profound ways in which sexual well-being contributes to a balanced life, advocating for a shift in perspective towards embracing our sexual selves.

One of the core aspects we've explored is the recognition that sexual health is far more than just the absence of dysfunction; it's about cultivating a fulfilling existence. This redefined understanding encourages us to view our sexuality not as a separate entity but as an intrinsic part of our overall well-being. By integrating these aspects, we create a more holistic approach to health, allowing us to flourish both individually and in our relationships.

The historical perspectives on desire illustrate how our understanding has evolved and shifted over millennia. From ancient societies that revered sexual energy to modern interpretations that occasionally stigmatise or suppress it, our attitudes have varied dramatically. We stand at a point where modern wisdom can draw lessons from the past, recognising sexual energy as a potent force for personal growth and transformation. Unlocking this knowledge empowers us to embrace our desires as natural, and ultimately beneficial, components of our human experience.

Science and exploration of the physiological and psychological underpinnings of sexual well-being have been enlightening. Understanding these elements offers clarity and validation to experiences that are often cloaked in mystery or misconception. By demystifying sexual health, we not only dispel myths but also provide the tools for individuals to harness sexual energy consciously and creatively.

Moreover, communication emerges as a pivotal skill in nurturing sexual health and achieving intimacy. Effective dialogue about desires and boundaries is essential in cultivating trust and understanding in relationships. By fostering open and respectful communication, we break down barriers, encourage mutual respect, and create environments where our sexuality can thrive unencumbered by judgement or alienation.

The multifaceted connections between nutrition, physical health, and sexual vitality serve as a reminder that our bodies are interconnected systems. Simple changes in diet and exercise can have profound impacts, rekindling desire and energy. These insights can stimulate a newfound appreciation for maintaining a lifestyle that supports all dimensions of our health, including our sexual lives.

As we've explored, each stage of life presents unique challenges and opportunities concerning sexual health. The narrative has often revolved around the potential for personal growth and adaptation. Young or aged, each phase asks us to reassess our needs and desires, pushing us to redefine what sexual fulfilment means on a personal level. The message is clear: sexual well-being is a lifelong journey, rich with potential for continual development and discovery.

Addressing the spiritual aspects of sexuality invites a broader understanding that transcends the physical and emotional realms. Many practices and philosophies underscore the unity of body, mind, and spirit, proposing that sexual energy can serve as a bridge between these areas. Such a holistic approach recharges not only how we interact with others but also how we connect within ourselves, fostering a sense of completeness and harmony.

The role of community and the importance of shared experiences underscore the need for supportive environments. By surrounding ourselves with allies and advocates, we can navigate our sexual journeys in safe, inclusive spaces. These communities act as vital networks of acceptance and growth, enhancing our understanding and practice of sexual wellness.

As we conclude, it remains essential to acknowledge the importance of embracing change and growth. Being open to learning and adapting—whether through shifting life stages or personal explorations—enhances our capacity for a richer life experience. This adaptability nurtures resilience, allowing us to respond dynamically to the evolving needs of our sexual health and well-being.

In embracing all these dimensions—historical, physiological, emotional, and spiritual—we lay the groundwork for achieving sexual synergy. This synthesis of knowledge and practice enables us to integrate sexual health seamlessly into our daily lives. As a result, we create a harmonious balance where health and desire complement each other, fostering a fulfilling life that honours our holistic existence. Through intentional practice and mindful living, the vibrancy of sexual well-being unfolds as an art, one that enriches our journey across the spectrum of human experience.

Appendix A:
Appendix

In bringing together the myriad insights and strategies explored throughout this book, the Appendix serves as a beacon for further exploration and personal empowerment. Here, readers will find a carefully curated selection of resources and exercises—tools designed to deepen their understanding and encourage the practical application of sexual wellness in everyday life. Whether you're seeking academic articles, books for pleasure reading, or a structured set of practices to enhance your sexual vitality, this section offers guidance tailored to a diverse set of interests and needs. It's a call to those striving for growth, encouraging a deeper dive into both personal and shared experiences of sexual health. As you integrate these learnings into your life, remember that each step you take towards embracing your sexuality is a step towards a more balanced, fulfilling existence. Let these resources fuel your journey towards self-discovery and holistic well-being, as you continue to explore and redefine your personal narrative of sexual vitality.

Resources for Further Reading

For those who are on a continuous journey to understanding and integrating their sexual health, expanding one's knowledge can be both empowering and enlightening. Whether you're delving into ancient philosophies, contemporary studies, or simply looking for effective practices, the range of literature available is vast and varied. In today's world, knowledge is more accessible than ever; yet, discerning which resources best fit your needs can sometimes be overwhelming.

One of the seminal works in the realm of sexuality and well-being is the trio of books by Emily Nagoski. Her exploration into the intricacies of sexual desire and health offers invaluable insights. Her books not only unravel the complexities of human arousal and emotional connectivity but also provide practical strategies to foster intimacy and self-awareness. These are essential readings for anyone wanting to bridge the gap between emotional wellness and sexual expression.

Diving into the historical perspectives, Thomas Laqueur's work on the history of sexuality can be an eye-opener. It captures how the understanding and interpretation of sexual desire have evolved across centuries. His research is comprehensive, painting a vivid picture of the societal norms and beliefs that have shaped modern perspectives. This resource is particularly beneficial for those who wish to comprehend how past constructs influence current societal norms and personal beliefs.

Within the scope of emotional and psychological well-being, Brene Brown's publications offer an exploration into the realm of vulnerability and shame, which are often closely interlinked with sexual health. By understanding emotional blocks that can hinder sexual expression, readers can learn to cultivate healthier relationships with themselves and others. Her work is a motivational approach to embracing one's imperfections and using them as a pathway to greater intimacy and connection.

An understanding of the physiological aspect of sexual health can be deepened through the work of Masters and Johnson, pioneers in exploring human sexual response. Their studies laid the foundation for much of today's research and clinical practice involving sexual function. Studying their findings can illuminate the physiological processes behind arousal and orgasm, shedding light on areas often shrouded in mystery and misinformation.

If you're interested in the intersection of fitness and sexual health, "The Science of Exercise" by John J. Ratey will be a valuable companion. This book outlines how physical activity can significantly influence sexual vitality. With information rooted in neuroscience, Ratey shares how regular exercise not only improves physical health but also boosts libido by enhancing mood, confidence, and overall mental well-being.

The role of hormones in sexual health is another crucial area. Aviva Romm's writings on balancing hormones through lifestyle choices and natural remedies offer an integrated approach to managing one's sexual health. Her methods provide practical advice on aligning physical and sexual health without relying heavily on pharmaceuticals, aligning closely with holistic health practices.

When examining the spiritual aspects of sexuality, Mantak Chia's teachings on Taoist sexual practices offer a fascinating perspective. His works delve into harnessing sexual energy as a powerful force for spiritual growth and personal health. Chia's teachings present a balance between ancient practices and modern needs, guiding readers on how to cultivate sexual energy to enhance both body and mind.

For an engaging and innovative look into therapy and sexual well-being, consider Esther Perel's transformative approach. Her insights into the importance of maintaining desire within long-term relationships challenge mainstream notions about commitment and passion. By acknowledging the delicate dance between intimacy and autonomy, Perel's work encourages readers to rethink traditional relationship dynamics and foster ongoing desire and connection.

Lastly, on the topic of sexual identity and inclusivity, works by bell hooks offer a powerful feminist perspective. Advocating for love and positivity in the face of enduring societal challenges, hooks challenges readers to consider how societal structures influence personal identity and relationship dynamics. Her voice is vital for anyone seeking understanding in a world that continually negotiates the complex interactions between power, vulnerability, and sexual health.

While these resources offer a foundational layer of understanding, it's crucial that each individual introspects and chooses materials that resonate with their personal path and experiences. The journey to integrating sexual health into overall well-being is deeply personal, and these readings serve as stepping stones in this enlightening voyage.

Exercises and Practices for Enhancing Sexual Well-being

Embarking on a journey towards enhanced sexual well-being involves a blend of introspection, physical practice, and emotional exploration. The exercises and practices in this section aim to deepen your connection with your sexual self, promoting an enriched sense of overall well-being. By incorporating these into your routine, you're not just nourishing your sexual health, but embracing a more balanced, fulfilling life.

One of the foundational practices for improving sexual well-being is the art of mindfulness. Mindfulness involves being present and fully engaged in the moment without judgment. This practice can help you become more aware of your body's sensations, desires, and boundaries, fostering a deeper connection with yourself. It could be as simple as dedicating five minutes a day to focus on your breathing, noticing how each breath fills and leaves your body. This kind of attentive presence can enhance your sensitivity to pleasure, making intimate experiences more fulfilling.

Trailblazing a path of physical vitality is crucial when assessing sexual well-being. Regular physical activity not only benefits your physical health but also improves libido and enhances sexual performance. Engaging in cardiovascular exercises like running, swimming, or cycling increases blood flow, which is vital for sexual function. Strength training exercises, on the other hand, enhance stamina, ensuring that you have the endurance to enjoy prolonged intimate moments. Additionally, activities like yoga and Pilates work on flexibility and strength, often targeted at the core and pelvic floor muscles. A stronger pelvic floor not only supports better control and intensity of orgasm but also aids in preventing sexual dysfunction.

The practice of *Kegel exercises* deserves special mention. Named after Dr. Arnold Kegel, these exercises target the pelvic floor muscles and can be done by anyone, regardless of gender. They involve contracting and releasing the pelvic floor muscles in sets, which can be performed discreetly anywhere. Regularly practicing Kegels can lead to improved bladder control, stronger orgasms, and heightened sexual pleasure. Finding time to incorporate these into your daily routine can bring about significant benefits over time.

Exploring intuitive movement through dance or expressive body movement can be an inspiring way to connect with your sexual energy. Not only does dance serve as a fun physical activity, but it also provides an avenue for self-expression and emotional release. Allowing your body to move freely can help shed inhibitions, increase confidence, and facilitate a more profound acceptance of your body. Try different styles - from salsa to belly dancing - and see what resonates with your spirit. Such practices encourage a playful yet powerful embrace of one's own sexuality.

Self-exploration is another pivotal aspect. Taking time to explore your own body without the external pressure of pleasing a partner can lead to a better understanding of what brings pleasure and satisfaction. This could be achieved through self-massage, which allows you to discover erogenous zones and areas that may heighten your experience of pleasure. The aim is to become in tune with your body's unique responses, deepening your understanding of what feels right for you.

Developing communication skills is equally important. Open and honest communication with your partner can greatly enhance sexual well-being. This practice isn't just about sharing your desires; it involves listening and responding to your partner's needs as well. Establishing a safe space for dialogue about intimacy can dissolve barriers and foster a deeper emotional connection. It also encourages mutual exploration, leading to richer and more fulfilling sexual experiences.

Artistic pursuits can also ignite and sustain sexual wellbeing. Engage in creative activities such as painting, writing, or playing music. These can serve as conduits for expressing facets of your sexuality that may remain unvoiced. The creative process helps not only in externalising internal feelings but also in realising previously undiscovered aspects of oneself. This kind of self-discovery fuels confidence and enthusiasm in all areas of life, including the sexual.

Exploration of sensuality through meditation is an enriching practice. Sensual meditation often involves visualising scenarios or environments that evoke sexual energy and peace. This practice sharpens your awareness of bodily sensations and pleasures, strengthening the mind-body connection. By dedicating time to this every week, you can cultivate a sense of calm and confidence that permeates into your intimate life.

Another worthwhile exploration is engaging with literature and resources that broaden your understanding of sexuality. There's an abundance of books, articles, and online courses dedicated to different aspects of sexual health and well-being. Not only can these resources provide valuable insights and techniques, but they can also challenge existing misconceptions and encourage open-mindedness.

It's important to remember that experimenting with these exercises and practices should be done with a sense of curiosity and openness. There's no single path that ensures enhanced sexual well-being for everyone, so find what resonates with you and your life circumstances. Trust in the journey and remain flexible to adapt and evolve as your understanding of yourself deepens.

Ultimately, the practices highlighted here are just steps on a journey to integrating sexual health as part of your overall well-being. They encourage a fuller appreciation for the pleasures of life and the powerful link between sexuality and personal health. By actively engaging with these practices, you're investing in a more harmonious and satisfying life journey, where sexual health plays a vital role in overall balance and happiness.

www.ingramcontent.com/pod-product-compliance
Lightning Source LLC
Chambersburg PA
CBHW020414290526
45785CB00002B/564